# the blood type diet cookbook

# the blood type diet cookbook

## Karen Vago & Lucy Degrémont

Over 100 fresh & delicious recipes
to transform your health & your life!

Thorsons

Thorsons
An Imprint of HarperCollins*Publishers*
77–85 Fulham Palace Road,
Hammersmith, London W6 8JB

The Thorsons website address is:
www.thorsons.com

and *Thorsons*
are trademarks of
HarperCollins*Publishers* Limited

First published by Thorsons 2001

10 9 8 7 6 5 4 3 2 1

A catalogue record of this book is
available from the British Library

ISBN 0 00 712795 2

Printed and bound in Great Britain by
Martins the Printers Ltd, Berwick upon Tweed

To Madeleine where all started and to Pauline,
Philip and Thomas where all continues

*Lucy Degrémont*


To Michel

*Karen Vago*

# acknowledgements

We wish to thank Dr Peter J. D'Adamo for his inspiring work in this field. In 1996 we read *Eat Right for Your Type*. This confirmed our intuitive natural choices: Lucy, blood type A, had been making her own tofu over the years, while Karen, blood type O, secretly enjoyed red meat despite the overall recommendations to avoid it. In 1998 our interest was further stimulated with *Cook Right for Your Type*. In 2001 the long awaited *Live Right for Your Type* appeared, extending blood type knowledge into a much larger spectrum.

Our thanks also go to Celia Wright, director of Higher Nature; Wanda Whiteley, our editor at Thorsons; Teresa Chris, our literary agent; Jillian Stewart; Sheila and Julian More and Burga and Fergus Belanger. Lastly, we wish to thank all those who allowed us to use their case histories of how the blood type diet changed their lives.

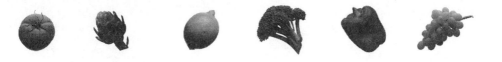

# contents

# foreword

This book has taken a long time to come to fruition. Over the years the idea behind it gradually blossomed, shaped by our observations of both gourmet cook books and health cook books. We felt there was a gap between the two aspects of eating – pleasure and health. We hope this book will bridge that gap.

Twenty years ago we were young mothers, each with three children, and in both our families one child had severe allergy problems. This motivated us to find curative solutions: one of them being nutrition. Our interest duly kindled, we went on to study nutrition (Karen) and gourmet cuisine (Lucy).

Shared passions have led to shared knowledge and during the past three years we have become increasingly interested in the science of eating according to one's blood group. Members of our families, friends and patients have all been reaping the benefits of this fundamental research, brought to light by Dr Peter D'Adamo. The results we have witnessed have been truly amazing and we feel privileged to be sharing this knowledge and our experience through these recipes.

For the past four seasons we have regularly left our respective family lives for cooking sessions in the Loire valley. We spent time with the producers of goat's cheese, we followed the aroma of summer strawberries to the fields where they were grown, we visited a small organic yogurt plant surrounded by big yellow sunflowers. We went completely over the top during the wild game season and marinated, stuffed and roasted everything from deer to partridges. We gathered fruit from the trees, little yellow plums to large pear-sized quinces, hazelnuts and walnuts. The days flew by in planning, shopping, researching, creating, measuring, cooking, writing, eating and sharing our food. We did it all ourselves and loved every minute of it.

Each season directed the choice of produce we used for our recipes as we feel nature provides chronobiologically what we need: in the summer friends gave us vegetables from their gardens, and in the autumn fruits from their trees and game from their forests. We believe in cooking with the freshest possible produce, using plenty of vegetables, fruit, free-range poultry, wild game (which by essence is organic), meat without hormones, wild fish if possible, herbs, spices and the finest quality oils.

Our recipes cover a wide range and include soups, salads, vegetables, goat's cheese, fish, poultry and game, meat, tofu and tempeh, sauces, desserts, drinks, festive dishes, Christmas and basic recipes. Each recipe is accompanied by blood type recommendations and, where appropriate, scientifically tested and traditionally proven dietary information about one of the main ingredients.

Tempting as it may be to jump straight in and try the recipes, do read the following chapter on blood types first. This provides background information on the origin of blood types, how our blood type can affect our health and how it interacts with the food we eat. Food recommendations are also given and these are complemented by the food lists, which provide a further guide on what each blood group should and should not eat.

To get you started we have created one week of menus for each season and for each blood type. In addition we felt it useful for you to have seven days of menus appropriate for all blood types. This will allow you to occasionally feed all blood groups at your table. The menus can be found at the back of the book, along with the recipe list that allows you to tell, at a glance, which recipe is suitable for which blood type. And for anyone still unsure of the benefits of following the diet we have included case histories for each blood type – these real life experiences are from patients who have experienced the turnaround in health that comes with following the blood type diet.

We trust that you will get pleasure from shopping and choosing the freshest foods in your markets and stores, enjoy the cooking process and savour the dishes you create. Lastly we believe you should leave the table feeling well nourished but with no heaviness in the stomach, and safe in the knowledge that what you just ate is on its way to building a healthy body and balanced mind. Enjoying that light, healthy feeling is our aim.


Good health and happy eating.

Karen Vago and Lucy Degrémont
Paris, September 2001

# 13 tips for a healthy body

1   Breathe in clean air. Oxygen is our first nutrient.
2   Drink plenty of natural or filtered water.
3   Eat according to your blood type.
4   Eat plenty of vegetables and fruit.
5   Choose organic meat, where available.
6   Choose wild fish rather than farmed fish as much as possible.
7   Avoid eating in a stressful situation. Wait for a calmer time.
8   Chew your food well. Deal with each mouthful before adding another one.
9   Add supplements when appropriate to deal with a deficiency, a health issue and for prevention.
10  Give priority to managing your stress level. If necessary consult a nutritional practitioner who can help strengthen your adrenal glands.
11  Exercise both in and outdoors.
12  Live with happy thoughts.
13  Each day allow yourself quiet moments on your own.

# the four blood
# types made easy

One of the most important aspects of health is the food we put in our bodies. Until recently, recommendations for food choices have mainly been based on the nutritional content of foods: how much of a particular vitamin or mineral does it contain, what is the fibre content, are the essential fatty acids unadulterated? Another trend has been to point an accusing finger at meat, whilst encouraging a greater consumption of grains. In my practice as a nutritionist, I have seen many type O patients for whom this type of macrobiotic diet has been a catastrophe. Relief was their understandable reaction on being told that not only was it okay for them to eat meat, but necessary if they wanted to be in good health. So should we be vegetarians or carnivores, follow the macrobiotic or paleolithic diet? What about the Mediterranean way of eating? However, the answer to the question of which diet suits us lies in who we are and not in what the diet is. What we eat interacts with each of us in a very particular way and that relationship is governed by our genetic makeup.

A food is not healthy or unhealthy *per se*. It interacts with us in a healthy or unhealthy manner. The work of Doctors James and Peter D'Adamo has enabled millions of people around the world to experience this. Peter D'Adamo has done a colossal job of furthering the findings of his father, Dr James D'Adamo: namely that your blood type (O, A, B or AB) is the key to what you should eat.

## How Did These Findings Come About?

Dr James D'Adamo, a naturopathic physician, observed that while some people did well on the typical vegetarian diet recommended in renowned European health spas, others did not. Following this initial observation he spent many years trying different diets on each of his patients until eventually he surmised that there must be something in our blood that determines what we should be eating. Little by little, food choices according to ABO blood typing became obvious. Those with blood type A, it seemed, benefited from a virtually meat-free diet with protein provided by soya and fish, while Os did well on a meat-based diet that avoided grains and milk products. These findings set the stage for his son's later scientific scrutiny.

Peter D'Adamo, a naturopathic physician in the making at that time (1980s), took advantage of university requirements to undertake research – and naturally he chose his father's field. What he was looking for was any information that could connect blood types to certain diseases, and if such information would give any weight to his father's ideas. Sure enough there it was. The prevalence of stomach cancer in blood type A was related to low gastric acid. This could explain why As should avoid meat – they did not produce enough gastric acid, which is essential for the complete digestion of animal protein. There was also relevant information on blood type O. This blood group is more prone to gastric ulcers – a condition usually caused by a highly acidic environment in the stomach. As James D'Adamo had discovered years before, Os could and should eat meat because they have the necessary acidic environment in the stomach to digest it properly.

This was just the beginning of the ongoing research into the relationship between ABO blood types and disease, and how selecting the right foods and living the right life can protect you.

## Human Evolution and Blood Types

The four different blood types, O, A, B and AB, didn't appear on earth all at the same time. The first three are a product of human evolution and the latter the consequence of As and Bs intermingling.

Man as we know him today appeared on this planet around 40,000BC, in eastern Africa. A branch of anthropology that investigates humankind's biological differences has concluded that our ancestors and the first men on earth, the hunter-gatherers, were blood type O. All mankind at that time, and for approximately the next 20,000 years, had the same blood type. Around 20,000BC a combination of increased population and depleted hunting grounds forced the hunter-gatherers to migrate to western Africa and the Asian and European continents. As our hunter ancestors adapted their diet and lifestyle to a different environment, their body also underwent a radical change. A new blood type appeared in response to a new man: the farmer. He cultivated grains, reared animals and lived in communities. Type A evolved from type O.

It was another 5,000–10,000 years before another blood type made its appearance as an evolutionary step from the original blood type O: type B. This appears to have been the result of hunter-gatherers migrating from the heat of eastern Africa to the cold conditions in the Himalayas, where Bs are thought to have evolved. These people were either nomads roaming the country to conquer better lands or farmers working the land they had settled on.

Blood type AB, only about 5 per cent of the world population, is the result of marriages between blood type A populations and blood type B populations. This blood type seems to have appeared not much more than 1,000 years ago.

What does all this tell us? Simply that blood groups are not arbitrary – they appeared as a direct response to man's physical and nutritional environment and those early blueprints laid down for each blood type continue to have relevance to this day.

## Our Blood Type is Part of Our Identity

Genetics have a lot to say as to who we are. The environment in which we live, our lifestyle and our thoughts may be even more important, but our blood type is part of our genetic design and cannot be ignored. The way we plan our life in terms of nutrition, exercise, thought, stress management etc. will make our blood type friend or foe. In other words, if we follow the recommendations that enable our body to positively adjust its biochemistry, we are likely to benefit from vibrant health. On the contrary, if we make choices that disrupt our metabolism, clog up our system with toxins and make our cells stick together, we are heading for trouble.

Our blood type gives information to our body, telling it how to react when confronted by a host of circumstances such as stress; invasion by viral, bacterial, parasitic or fungal infections; or food entering the body. Psychologically and physically each blood group reacts differently to these influences: a specific food can be beneficial or detrimental to our health depending on whether we are an O, an A, a B or an AB; an infective agent will have something to hold onto depending on our blood group; our susceptibility to common diseases or more serious ones is linked to our blood group; the means by which an O will lose weight is not the same as for an A.

And this isn't anecdotal information. Much of this information can be found in scientific literature. Dr D'Adamo has referenced over 1500 research studies to back up his work.

## My Personal Experience with the Blood Type Diet

As a nutritionist I ate, for many years, what I considered to be a very healthy diet – at least I thought it was. I was cutting down on red meats and increasing fish and poultry, replacing wheat with other grains such as rye and spelt (in bread), eating rice, quinoa and millet. I made the effort to cook lentils and pulses. Instead of cow's cheese I would eat goat's and sheep's cheese and yogurt. I was taking plenty of supplements, as well as digestive enzymes. Yet despite all this I still struggled with my weight and had trouble with my immune system during the winter.

Then one day I came across a paragraph on "Blood type and diet" in Dr Ralph Golan's book, *Optimal Wellness*. This very briefly described Peter D'Adamo's work, and to me it sounded so right. Being an O, something deep down in me had always resisted becoming a vegetarian. I just instinctively knew I needed animal protein.

I applied the little I read in Ralph Golan's description to myself and soon began to feel the benefit. Suitably impressed, I put into practice the advice in Peter D'Adamo's book. The result? I moved onto a higher level of health. Being blood type O I had permission to eat meat, which I love. Unfortunately I had to give up cheese (which is particularly difficult when you live in France). Os can only have a small amount of goat's and sheep's cheese (I was still eating too much). Grains are to be avoided and I can attest to that. Whenever I was tempted to eat normal wheat bread or even too much spelt bread, I immediately felt the difference – a heaviness set in and I put on weight. That was when I first started the diet – I now know what to do to feel good, be healthy and lean. If I am tempted all I need to do is remind myself of how good I feel and, more often than not, following the blood type diet takes precedence over the indulgence. Although it took a little time to adjust to some of the changes, I now positively enjoy the many beneficial foods that are suitable for my blood type.

Since discovering Peter D'Adamo's book, I have introduced his findings to my patients and continue to do so. To me, the most convincing evidence that there is truth in the blood type diet lies in my own experience and the results my patients are getting with this method of eating.

# the key to the blood type diet: lectins

Extensively researched for their good and bad effects, but little spoken of in nutritional circles, lectins encountered in the foods we eat are the so-called "scientific link between blood type and diet". Before looking into the effects lectins can have in our bodies, let me give a brief description of what knowing about your blood type means – other than making sure you don't receive the wrong blood during a transfusion.

## the reality of lectins

How does our blood type influence our food choices? The main reason is the presence of lectins in the vegetable and animal kingdom. They can also be found in micro-organisms and viruses. Basically lectins are a type of protein. Not all foods contain lectins but those we encounter in our foods are of great importance to our health.

The beneficial and harmful effects of lectins are being extensively studied. It has been found, for example, that the lectins in the following foods have beneficial effects: the lectin in the edible snail has an anti-cancer effect in types A and AB, peanuts may have a preventive effect against breast cancer in blood type A, and lentils and broad (fava) beans may also have anti-cancer effects in type A.

The harmful lectins should, in contrast, be considered our number one enemy. You will soon understand why. Lectins are like mischievous little underworld creatures. They come along in the body, seek out the cells they are akin to, make them clump together so they are stuck and can't carry out their work properly, then run off to do the same elsewhere. Or in the words of Dr D'Adamo, "Once the intact

lectin protein settles someplace in your body, it literally has a magnetic effect on
the cells in that region. It clumps the cells together and they are targeted for
destruction, as if they too were foreign invaders."

Any system of the body can be affected, be it the nervous, digestive, cardiovascular or hormonal system. Lectins are proteins that can bind to any molecule with
a sugar portion on the surface of its cells. And precisely the way our blood type is
expressed is through the presence of specific sugars on the surface of our cells. It so
happens that many lectins are blood type specific, meaning that they will be
attracted to body cells of one blood type and not necessarily those of another. The
word lectin comes from the Latin for "to choose", describing an essential characteristic of these proteins. They choose, according to blood type, the cells that they are
going to work on, making them agglutinate. These cells can be red blood cells,
white blood cells, cells of the gastrointestinal tract, the pancreas, the kidneys, the
liver … but the first cells met by lectins are, of course, those of the digestive tract.
That is where they make their first impact. According to researcher Arpad Pusztai,
the lectins in our diet have an enormous influence on the way our digestive tract is
going to respond to the foods it comes in contact with and this, in turn, affects our
health in general. I have noticed that digestive symptoms improve in the first days
of following the blood type diet. My patients feel less bloated, have fewer spasms,
less nausea, and they find food doesn't lie as heavy on the stomach.

Dietary lectins can have an effect on different aspects of digestion. They can
inactivate certain digestive enzymes and damage the gut wall, thus impairing
absorption. This can also lead to substances that would normally remain in the gut
leaking through the gut wall into the general circulation – a condition referred to as
leaky gut. When the lining of the small intestine cannot act as an efficient barrier
any longer bacteria, food antigens capable of triggering an allergic-type reaction in
the body, and toxins, can all cross into the bloodstream. Joint inflammation,
rheumatoid arthritis and ankylosing spondylitis have all been linked with gut per-
meability. Lectins can also cause painful inflammation of the gut lining.

It has been found that 5–10 per cent of the lectins in food can pass into the bloodstream and circulate in the body. There they can cause inflammatory reactions such
as arthritis and allergies; disrupt thyroid hormone (hypo and hyper thyroidism) and
insulin production (diabetes); interfere with the normal function of the nervous system; and settle in the kidneys and the liver, disrupting their function.

The process of digestion can affect lectins in various ways. Lectins are usually
not inactivated by gastric acids, meaning they will reach the intestine intact.
Chewing can actually aggravate some lectin activity. Cooking also has varying
effects on lectins. Certain bean lectins are inactivated by specific soaking and
cooking procedures (see instructions on page 188), while the negative aspects of
other lectins are increased by cooking (bananas are one example). Interestingly,
the lectin contained in wheat – a grain that so many people need to avoid – is inactivated by the process of sprouting.

The main reason for avoiding specific foods on the blood type diet is the presence of lectins. A second reason for avoidance is the responsibility a food may have for the higher incidence of certain health problems in each blood type. For example, blood type A has a higher incidence of cardiovascular disease associated with higher levels of cholesterol. As a protective measure olive oil – which has beneficial effects on cholesterol levels – should be consumed rather than butter. A third reason for avoidance is the internal makeup, the blood group individuality so to speak, that determines which food or food group should be avoided. For example, Os have a problem dealing with milk products and should avoid them almost totally.

Using various laboratory and clinical methods Dr D'Adamo and his team have tested the foods covered in this book and their effects on the body. As the research into blood type diets is an ongoing process it is wise to always seek the latest information. Peter D'Adamo's website www.dadamo.com is a rich source of information for the layperson, the practitioner and the researcher.

I urge you to read all of the following information, rather than just that on your particular blood type, as some of the health advice is relevant to all types.

# the four blood types: food requirements and health characteristics

## blood type o: general food recommendations

Humanity's ancestors were all blood type O. The hunter-gatherers ate what they could find growing or roaming in their environment. Their diet was composed of meat, fish, fowl, leaves, roots, berries, fruits, seeds and nuts. These are, in general, the foods you will do best on if you are blood type O. Eat plenty of vegetables with meat, fish and fowl – your best sources of protein. Include nuts and seeds (particularly linseeds and walnuts) several times a week as these provide extra protein, essential fatty acids and some minerals. Fruit – both dried and fresh – is a good way of satisfying your natural need for something sweet.

### Meat, Poultry and Game

Do not worry about eating meat – it is good for you because your body is genetically made to metabolise it. Your digestive system normally has the necessary acids in the stomach and enzymes in the intestines to digest animal protein and fat. However, if you are not accustomed to eating animal protein you may need to gradually introduce meat in small quantities and take digestive enzymes for a while.

Eating meat for you is essential as it will balance your blood sugar levels and help to counteract cravings for carbohydrates. Having good steady energy levels and not making fat from sugar depends on your consumption of animal protein.

Maintaining and building good healthy muscle mass also depends on eating animal
protein, and this will contribute to your being lean. Choose quality organic meat as
often as possible. Red meat is your best protein choice. Avoid pork. A recommendation to eat meat does not mean, however, that you can eat huge amounts of it –
have no more 3½–6oz/100–180g of meat or poultry six to eight times a week.

# Tamara

Blood Type O
Age 27

I became ill towards the end of 2000. The symptoms were very diffuse (muscle ache,
skin rashes), but pointed towards some kind of auto-immune disease. My disease was
never properly diagnosed and in the end the doctors bade me farewell without giving
me any treatment. At this point I decided to turn to alternative medicine. I should add
that for one year prior to my becoming ill, I had been following a vegan diet.

I consulted with Karen, and on her advice I have been eating according to my blood
type (O) and taking a variety of supplements for about six months. The effect on my
condition has been dramatic. I feel fitter and my energy level has risen. I have experienced an improvement in my sleep patterns and in my daily exercise routine (jogging).
The most salient effect has been as a result of giving up wheat flour – I feel a great deal
lighter and seem to be digesting other flours (eg. rye and spelt) a lot better. To cut a long
story short, I feel light as a feather and healthy.

## Seafood

You are the only blood type who can eat virtually all shellfish: oysters, crab, lobster,
shrimp, clams etc. Enjoy these whenever you can. Your choice of fish is also large.
Fatty fish are especially good for you, as they contain beneficial omega-3 oils that
counter inflammation.

## Vegetables

All blood types benefit from eating plenty of vegetables. They are the basis of a
healthy diet. Ensure they are as fresh as possible and eat them every day for lunch
and dinner – raw or cooked, juiced, in salads, in soup – and as a snack. You will find
information about the tremendous benefits of eating these health-giving plants in
the recipe section. Green leafy vegetables such as kale, spring greens (collards),
turnip greens and dandelion leaves should be included often as they provide much-
needed calcium. Os should avoid potatoes, but you can replace them with sweet
potatoes. If you feel leafy vegetables are not filling enough, add a second vegetable

such as celeriac, parsnips, kohlrabi, pumpkin, beetroot (beet), carrots, fresh green peas, instead of adding the traditional potato or rice accompaniment. We tend to forget that grains are not the only food that contain carbohydrates; so too do vegetables. And the carbohydrates provided by vegetables are better for you than those derived from grains.

## Fruits

Vegetables and fruits are similar in their nutrient content. They are our best source of vitamins, minerals, phytonutrients and antioxidants. Fruits generally have a higher sugar content than vegetables. However, this comes in the form of fructose, which raises blood sugar levels much less rapidly than sucrose – the sugar found in table sugar and refined carbohydrates such as white flour. This is an important difference. Fruit can help maintain balanced energy levels, while refined sugars can make them fluctuate wildly.

If you wish to lose weight eat a piece of fruit 30 minutes before your meals. This practice has been shown to moderate appetite and encourage weight loss.

Not all fruits are suitable for Os. You should, for instance, avoid kiwi, oranges, certain melons and coconuts.

# Bruno

Blood Type O
Age 37

I am a former high-level racing cyclist. After reaching 30 I began experiencing health problems: my weight began to increase, my digestion became a concern, and I experienced backache. I tried various diets and health recommendations and although I lost weight, I would simply regain it.

Around this time I met Karen, who recommended the blood type diet. Dr D'Adamo's book was not yet available in France, but just a few months later I discovered it by chance (although I do not believe in pure chance!) and that triggered my seriously following the diet.

I lost 28kg (61lb) in nine months, but to me the most important benefit has been an increased energy level. I am now in wonderful shape and have started racing again. I am scoring excellent results and recently won a race against a team of younger cyclists. If I go off my diet my body is quick to remind me of my misdemeanour. If, for example, I have a cup of coffee before a race I get cramps in my legs.

## Nuts, Seeds and their Oils

Nuts and seeds should be a regular part of your diet. They are a source of essential fatty acids, protein and minerals. I consider the most valuable ones to be walnuts and flaxseeds (linseeds). Walnuts contain linolenic acid, a valuable omega-3 fatty acid rare in our modern diets. Eat freshly-cracked walnuts and use walnut oil in salads, but do not cook with it. If you heat it, the valuable fatty acid will be damaged. Flaxseeds are a very valuable seed, much used by practitioners of natural medicine. They contain lignans that are transformed in the gut into substances that have anti-cancer effects and that can regulate hormone levels during the menopause or in cases of premenstrual syndrome. Its essential oil, linolenic acid, has anti-inflammatory effects (type Os have a tendency toward inflammatory conditions) that relieve symptoms of rheumatoid arthritis, eczema, psoriasis, etc. Flaxseeds have also been shown to reduce cholesterol levels and coronary heart disease. They also contain a mucilage that is very effective against constipation.

I recommend that my patients make regular use of walnuts and flaxseeds and their oils. A convenient way of eating flaxseeds is to grind them in an electric coffee grinder (cleaned first, of course!) and sprinkle 1–3 tablespoons on salads or stir through yogurt or apple sauce. Always choose cold pressed oils, as these retain their fatty acids intact. The only cold pressed oil that withstands the heat of cooking is olive oil. Use the other recommended oils for your blood type in salads.

# Monika

Blood Type O
Age 53

Before trying the blood type diet I had been suffering from constipation, a white tongue and pain in my arms and legs for 10 years. I had been taking herbal infusions and plant supplements with no significant improvement. On consulting a naturopath I was also advised to include cheese and grains in my daily meals. I followed this regime for several years but my problems persisted.

When I met Karen her first question was: "What is your blood type?" Like many others I was surprised to hear that my blood type could have a bearing on my diet. After giving her my meal plans she said "wheat and milk products are not for you". These were precisely the foods I included regularly in my meals. I also needed to eat red meat – something that I was previously advised to avoid. I followed the blood type diet and took appropriate supplements. The result? Just two months later I felt a substantial improvement. In addition, my cholesterol level – which was slightly elevated with my previous diet – is now well within the normal range.

### Grains

Grains should not be a regular part of your diet, although you do have a certain degree of tolerance for some types of grains. You can eat small amounts of rice, rye, millet, spelt, oats, kamut and buckwheat. Wheat, corn and barley (and for some, oats) can encourage weight gain. They are also very often held responsible for various inflammatory conditions such as arthritis and fibromyalgia. However, you can eat sprouted grains as in Essene bread (also called sprouted wheat bread). Although it is made with wheat, the sprouting process destroys the lectins that normally should be avoided. Essene bread is beneficial for all blood types.

## what is Essene bread?

The name Essene comes from a Jewish sect that lived in the time of Jesus Christ, and in the same region. The Essenians led a very austere life and believed in the importance of "live" food. They made a special kind of bread from sprouted grains that they baked, or rather dried, in the sun. Today Essene bread is baked in a slow oven. In France, Essene bread is made with sprouted wheat, rye, spelt or kamut. The consistency, appearance and taste bear little resemblance to normal bread. It is moist and slightly sweet. Handle with care because it tends to break. If you wish, you may lightly toast it; in this case it is best cut into thick slices. Among my patients some love this bread and others would much rather do without it. It is highly digestible and works wonders if you are constipated.

### Milk Products

Cheese and yogurt made from cow's milk, and cow's milk itself, should be avoided. Nevertheless you may eat goat's and sheep's cheese (2oz/60g) and yogurt once or twice a week. If you need to lose weight or suffer from any type of inflammatory disease such as asthma, eczema or arthritis, or if you have a tendency to produce mucous in the respiratory tract, avoid dairy products altogether until your condition has improved. You may then find your body is able to tolerate small amounts again.

If you are concerned about not getting enough calcium remember that cows do not drink milk and yet produce milk that is very rich in calcium. Where does it come from? From their vegetarian diet. Here are some foods that are good for your blood type and that contain more calcium, weight for weight, than whole milk: green leafy vegetables (collard leaves, kale, turnip leaves, dandelion greens), figs, almonds, sunflower seeds, kelp, dulse, tofu and watercress. Broccoli, sesame seeds and walnuts also contain good amounts. If you feel you are not getting sufficient calcium because you are not making these food choices often enough, it would be wise to take a calcium supplement. If you are pregnant or breast feeding definitely take a supplement.

## Legumes and lentils

The general tendency for several years now has been to recommend that people reduce their consumption of red meat and obtain more protein from vegetable sources. To provide complete protein, eating a combination of legumes and seeds, legumes and grains, or legumes and milk products was recommended. This, again, may seem good if you only consider nutrition from the point of view of the foods. If your blood type is O, this is definitely not a good way to get your protein. Your body needs meat – good lean organic meat, just like the kind your blood type ancestors ate. You can eat two or three portions of legumes a week but do not use them as a replacement for meat in your diet. You can also eat soya products such as tofu, but again do not rely on soya as a main source of protein.

---

# Anne

Blood Type O
Age 36

When I was diagnosed as having multiple sclerosis, I consulted a nutritionist on the advice of my osteopath. The food recommendations I was given were based on the blood type diet. By following this approach I didn't expect to heal myself but simply to reduce the negative effects that certain foods can have on the body.

I had been eating huge amounts of milk products, plenty of grains and very little vegetables and protein. I paid great attention to the quantities I was eating but was still having trouble controlling my weight. Almost every day I suffered from gas, bloating and constipation. I also regularly experienced an irrepressible need for sugar. Following the blood type diet has significantly changed my relationship with food. I have discovered the pleasure of choosing my food and cooking it. I feel much less tired in spite of my illness and medical treatment, and many of my symptoms have disappeared. The grey circles under my eyes have almost completely gone, and the texture of my skin has changed for the better.

I thought it would be difficult and constraining to follow this dietary discipline but little by little the desire to eat cakes and biscuits, sweets and rich meals has disappeared and I have rediscovered a healthy taste for food.

---

# type o: health issues

The blood type diet is not the answer to all ills and following it will not give you complete protection from disease. But it is a powerful means of setting the stage to allow your body to perform to the best of its ability. The basic ideas that underpin the blood type diet tie in very well with research being done into how nutrition influences the way our genes express themselves.

Our genes hold information as to whether an illness could assail our body or not. This information does not necessarily mean the illness will develop. It will if the correct conditions are present. It will not if conditions that prevent our genes from expressing that illness are present. Dr Jeffrey S. Bland has written a book about this concept, *Genetic Nutritioneering*. In a tribute to Dr D'Adamo he says, "It is truly fascinating that medicine is moving from a period of the past one hundred years when disease was considered to be 'hard wired' into our genes, to a time when we realize that we can play a role in strengthening our genetic inheritance through our daily living". The blood type diet does exactly this. "Eat right for your type" and you will strongly reduce your risk of having to deal with the potential health conditions hidden in your genes.

## Digestion

As you will have read in the previous section, lectins present in the foods you should avoid make their first impact in your digestive system. Digestive complaints such as those associated with irritable bowel syndrome – bloating, gas, pain, spasm, constipation and diarrhoea – are greatly reduced by following the blood type diet, and often disappear. If these complaints persist they are often due to an imbalanced bowel flora. In this case, consider taking a good probiotic supplement. These symptoms can also be caused by the presence of undesirable parasites, bacteria or yeast (candida for example). It may be necessary to check this with your doctor or a reputable diagnostic laboratory if the diet doesn't lessen or remove your symptoms.

As previously stated, type Os normally produce enough stomach acid to digest meat. However, if certain conditions occur simultaneously, such as too much stress and eating the wrong foods for your type, your stomach can produce *too much* acid. You may then suffer from heartburn or stomach ulcers. Following your diet recommendations should clear the condition. If this is not sufficient you may need to try a stress management program and some soothing herbs such as slippery elm, marshmallow or DGL (deglycyrrhizinated licorice root).

## Weight

Many of my overweight type O patients have experienced good weight loss results by following the diet and a dynamic exercise program. You needn't try any of those powders, shakes or pills to lose weight – just eat lean animal protein and plenty of vegetables. Wheat and milk products are largely responsible for weight gain in this blood type. I am living proof of this fact, my blood type being O.

Another weight loss-promoting habit is to eat a substantial breakfast, a mid-morning snack, a real meal at lunch, a mid-afternoon snack and an early and light dinner. A study has shown that people who ate their last daily meal late in the afternoon, rather than in the evening, lost weight. This was the only change they made in their eating habits.

Each time you eat make sure you include some form of protein. For breakfast you could have an egg or some fish, as well as some fruit (avoid cereal in any form). For lunch and dinner eat vegetables (cooked and/or raw) with fish, meat or poultry. Snacks should also have some form of protein – try nuts or yogurt (soya or sheep) with fruit. Avoid eating grains and cheese if you wish to lose weight.

Exercise is very important for this blood type. Vigorous exercise is what you need to get your body burning fat. Type Os have a tendency towards a sluggish metabolism if they do not force themselves through three to four 30-minute sessions of strenuous exercise each week. You will find it gives you a positive outlook on life and enables you to respond better to stress.

---

# Agathe

Blood Type O
Age 9

I wanted to see a nutritionist because I wanted to lose weight. But mostly I wanted to feel better. In my class nearly everyone weighed 39kg (85lb) and I weighed 10kg (22lb) more. When I saw them I said to myself: "If I could only be like them."

I visited a nutritionist with my mother and was given a food list that suited my blood type. When I saw the list I thought I could never do it, but I did it and I felt much better. I had a bowel movement every day, I drank water and I paid attention to what I ate. I felt my tummy was getting smaller and I was less tired. It really helped and I am happy.

---

## Thyroid

If you are exercising and following the diet and you still have difficulty losing weight, it is worthwhile checking your thyroid – a weak point for your O system. Hypothyroidism can also be responsible for chronic fatigue, weight gain and difficulty losing weight, depression, low libido, period problems in women, a weak immune system and many more symptoms. Here is an easy test you can do yourself. As soon as you wake up in the morning and before moving about, take your basal metabolic temperature. Place a traditional thermometer (not electronic) in

your armpit for 10 minutes, and remain quiet during this time. Follow this procedure at the same time on three consecutive days (menstruating women should do
this on days 2, 3 and 4 of their cycle). A temperature below 36.6°C (97.8°F) on three
consecutive days most probably indicates low thyroid function.

Blood tests alone do not always give enough information as to what your thyroid status is. If the blood test indicates low thyroid function, fine. If it is normal
according to the lab, then it is necessary to consider your symptoms and your temperature before dismissing low thyroid function. A practitioner who knows about
thyroid function would be able to help you determine whether your symptoms
point towards low thyroid function. I also recommend Martin Budd's book *Why am
I so Tired?* He has studied and treated hypothyroid problems for over 20 years.

## Inflammation

I find that type O patients with joint or muscle pain or any other type of inflammatory condition usually find relief within a few weeks of following the diet.
Inflammation is another weak spot in blood type O. This can be largely avoided if
you eat the right foods. The culprits are dairy products and grains. I have tested
this myself. Many years ago I strained my knee while on a skiing holiday. The
resulting pain lasted for several months then disappeared, only to reappear inter-
mittently for no apparent reason. However, since I stopped eating wheat my knee
has been fine. If I do make an exception and eat too much dairy produce or grain,
then I invariably feel a twinge in my knee again.

---

# Nathalie

Blood Type O
Age 27

For several months I had been feeling very tired; I also had a persistent tingling feeling
in my arms and legs, and my muscles were very weak. A medical examination revealed
inflammation in the cervical area of the spinal cord, and I was treated with intravenous
cortisol. That took care of the muscular problems. However, I was still very tired, still felt
a tingling in my hands and I had a very bad complexion.

My osteopath recommended that I see a nutritionist. I followed the blood type diet
to the letter and within two to three days I felt an improvement. My fatigue, irritability,
muscular problems and constipation have now gone. In addition, I have lost the weight
I had gained from months of inactivity.

---

# blood type a: general food recommendations

The hunter-gatherers were forced to migrate when the wild game that was their main food source became scarce. Unfortunately their proficiency at hunting was such that they soon found themselves in the same position in their new lands and they were forced to adapt to new living conditions. A new lifestyle and environment brought with it a new internal environment. Blood type A was born. The new type A man cultivated land and raised animals, and was far more suited to eating the products of his labour – namely grains.

What you can eat and thrive on today has a lot to do with past conditioning. Of the four blood types, type A is the closest to a vegetarian. Vegetarianism is not recommended for the other three blood groups, due to their inner makeup.

Your body likes fish; pulses (legumes) and lentils; tofu; fermented soya products such as tempeh, miso and natto; nuts and seeds; grains; fruit and of course plenty of vegetables. You should avoid cow's milk products, although it is okay to eat some goat and sheep products. Here is the general outline of what your diet should look like.

## Seafood

In the animal realm your best choice of foods comes from the sea. As you will read in the section on health issues for type As, you have a higher risk (along with type AB) of cardiovascular disease than Os and Bs. Fish offers protection from this. You can choose from a large selection of suitable fish but should avoid all shellfish. Make sure you regularly eat fatty fish such as mackerel, sardines, trout, salmon, herring etc. When you eat fish limit the quantity because your digestive makeup doesn't enable you to digest large amounts. However, you should be able to judge this for yourself once you learn to listen to your body's needs.

## Meat and Poultry

Your best choices of protein are determined by the fact that your stomach acid levels tend to be low. In order to properly digest animal protein we need ample amounts of hydrochloric acid. You are therefore better off eating only small amounts of chicken, turkey, guinea fowl and deriving most of your protein from soya products and fish. You may also include eggs in your diet. I have noticed that many of my blood type A patients adopted these choices before knowing about the blood type diet. These are usually patients who are already on the way to better health and have discovered by themselves what foods their body prefers. Eating meat will only clog up your system, make you feel sluggish and heavy, and add weight. Lucy (co-writer of this book) is an A, and knows all about this feeling.

## Legumes, Lentils and Soya Products

Pulses and lentils are another excellent source of protein for this blood group. They provide a good source of complex carbohydrates and fibre. All of the health benefits attributed to legumes apply to you more than to any other blood type. Legumes contain phytosterols and fibre that have cholesterol-lowering and cancer-protective effects (type As have a higher risk of cancer than some other blood types – this is discussed in greater detail on page 23). In addition, legumes encourage good bowel function, which protects against colon cancer and haemorrhoids. Fibre regulates both blood sugar levels and insulin sensitivity, thereby offering protection against diabetes.

Soya beans and other legumes have approximately the same qualities. However, soya beans, and hence soya products, have a higher fat content with plenty of essential fatty acids and also a higher protein content with an excellent amino acid profile. Soya is a good source of lecithin, which has been shown to lower cholesterol levels (As are at higher risk of elevated cholesterol) and help the liver and gall bladder function effectively.

Soya also contains phytoestrogens that exert both a mild estrogenic and anti-estrogenic effect. In other words these compounds have a balancing effect on the hormonal system.

---

# Robert

Blood Type A
Age 56

It is often under the recommendation of his wife that a man goes to see a nutritionist. Over the years I have increasingly suffered from digestive difficulties and painful joints. My professional life is intense and stressful but also enjoyable.

As a type A my food plan excluded meat and dairy. This was not easy but I was able to compensate with fish, which I like. After one month, with the help of some supplements, I regained digestive well-being and experienced a notable reduction in the pain in my joints.

As for the stress issue, I decided to do an adrenal stress test which revealed that my stress hormones, cortisol and DHEA, were high. I was told that since my DHEA was high, this would protect me for a time against the effects of high cortisol. However, I should avoid remaining in this state for too long as this could lead to tired adrenal glands in the end. To reduce my physiological stress response I take herbs and specific nutrients recommended by the nutritionist.

---

## Grains

In general type As can eat grains. However, you should limit your consumption of wheat and avoid wheat bran and wheat germ. Avoid wheat altogether if you have inflammatory problems such as arthritis and easy build-up of mucus in the respiratory tract. Wheat and corn can make some type As gain weight; in this case it is better to avoid these two grains.

Of all the blood groups you can enjoy grains most, but eat them in moderation. In our society we tend to eat too many grains and cereals – too much bread, pasta, cakes and cookies. They are a convenient and quick way of getting food in our systems: bread is quickly cut, pizza is easily stuck in the oven and pasta is cooked in no time. Many people eat these foods several times a week – if not every day – when they should be eating vegetables and healthy protein. So beware! Change your habits now for the sake of your health.

All this being said, grains do have health benefits. They complement legumes and the two provide all the amino acids needed to make up a complete protein. Legumes are low in the amino acids, methionine and cysteine; grains are low in lysine. Grains are a good source of fibre (although we tend to forget that vegetables are too), minerals and B vitamins.

You may eat sprouted grains, as sprouting destroys the lectins that normally should be avoided. Sprouted grain Essene bread is a particularly good source and is beneficial for all blood groups (for more information on Essene bread see page 10).

## Nuts and Seeds

These are another protein source that have the added benefit of fibre and minerals. Walnuts have a detoxifying effect in the intestines and are a good source of linolenic acid (omega-3 oil), a fatty acid lacking in our diet. Flaxseeds (linseeds) contain the highest amount of linolenic acid of all the seeds and are rich in lignans that, once converted in the intestines, have anti-cancer properties. The omega-3 oils are effective in lowering cholesterol levels and treating inflammatory conditions such as arthritis and eczema. Flaxseeds have been shown to improve women's hormonal cycles, increasing the progesterone/estrogen ratio and encouraging ovulation and healthy ovaries. Try grinding flaxseeds in an electric coffee grinder (cleaned of all traces of coffee). They can then be sprinkled on your food or you can also add them to a glass of water or juice. Keep them in the refrigerator for no longer than five days. Flaxseeds, ground or unground, are an excellent remedy for constipation. Peanuts, which are actually a legume, contain a lectin that may have anti-cancer properties. Include peanuts in your food choices. They are a good source of protein.

# Madeleine

Blood Type A
Age 88

At 85 I decided it was still not too late to seriously follow Dr D'Adamo's method of eating according to one's blood type. During most of my life I've suffered from allergy problems: runny nose, itchy eyes and, most often, a lack of energy. I had wondered at one time if wheat may have been the source of the problem, but convinced myself that it was unlikely.

I read and reread Dr D'Adamo's book *Eat Right 4 Your Type*. At first I was convinced that my blood group was type O since I felt I shared many of the characteristics that went with that blood type. I started cutting out wheat and most cereals and I felt better. Eventually I had a blood test which revealed to my surprise that I was type A. The difference in food choices between group O and group A made all the difference to my total feeling of well-being. I started cutting down on meat and adding more soya products to my meals. Along with my multi-vitamin, my health practitioner advised me to take an extra vitamin C and a vitamin B complex, and added vitamin $B_{12}$ plus some Gingko Biloba. From then on my stress response calmed down and I started sleeping soundly – this was new to me as I had not been sleeping well for years. I exercise daily outside (weather permitting), practise Qi Gong breathing and relaxation movements, garden, cord my wood, knit, read and get the best out of cable television. My life is very full.

Today, at 88, I feel so well, with a high energy level and a joy and enthusiasm for life. Giving up some favourite foods – even some fruit and vegetables – has been very worthwhile. It is always so good to hear friends greet me with "You look so well!"

## Milk Products

As with blood type O, milk products should only play a small part in your diet. You can, however, have a bit more than type Os. As is the case with all types, signs of excess mucus in the respiratory system should alert you to reducing your consumption. Cow's milk products are largely to be avoided. Goat's and sheep's milk products are better for you. However, nothing in this range of foods can be said to be beneficial. When you read about blood types B and AB you will see that they are the only groups that derive any benefit from milk products.

## Vegetables

All blood types benefit from eating plenty of vegetables. They are the basis of a healthy diet. Ensure they are as fresh as possible and eat them every day for lunch and dinner – raw or cooked, juiced, in salads, in soup – and as a snack. You will find information about the tremendous benefits of eating these health-giving plants in the recipe section. As you cannot count on milk products for your calcium, make calcium-rich, green leafy vegetables such as kale, spring greens (collards), turnip greens and dandelion leaves a regular part of your diet.

Avoid tomatoes as they contain a lectin that is detrimental to the type A system. When you make salad dressings, replace the commonly used vinegar with lemon juice. Your sensitive stomach lining will be grateful. Avoid all types of pepper. The best oils for salads are flaxseed, olive and walnut oils. Avoid cotton seed, peanut and corn oil. Give flavour to your dressings with fresh herbs, tamari (Japanese soy sauce) and plenty of garlic. If you have a problem digesting garlic this may mean your liver has difficulty doing its job as a detoxifier. In this case garlic isn't the problem, your liver is. See a nutritionist or naturopathic doctor to help sort this out.

## Fruits

Vegetables and fruits are similar in their nutrient content. They are our best source of vitamins, minerals, phytonutrients and antioxidants. Fruits generally have a higher sugar content than vegetables. However, this comes in the form of fructose, which raises blood sugar levels much less rapidly than sucrose – the sugar found in table sugar and refined carbohydrates such as white flour. This is an important difference. Fruit can help maintain balanced energy levels, while refined sugars can make them fluctuate wildly.

If you wish to lose weight eat a piece of fruit 30 minutes before your meals. This practice has been shown to moderate appetite and encourage weight loss.

Not all fruits are good for you. Oranges are too acidic for your sensitive stomach – many of my type A patients have noticed this on their own. You should also avoid tropical fruits such as bananas, guavas, mangoes, coconuts and papayas.

---

# Marie

Blood Type A
Age 58

The blood type diet appealed to me on an intellectual level. I realised that since childhood I had a very strong attraction and appetite for foods that I should be eating. I was happy to see this is actually being confirmed by a scientific approach to foods. I always had a repulsion for red meat.

If I go off the diet I immediately feel digestive and physical heaviness, abdominal and general bloatedness and it takes my body several days to eliminate the offending food. In the past I would go to seminars on personal development where the food that was served was vegetarian with plenty of wheat in its various forms. Invariably I would return home having put on 3kg. Now I know why.

---

**What Can I Drink?**

Water, water, water. *Your Body's Many Cries for Water* is a fascinating book written by Dr F. Batmanghelidj about the many signals of thirst that are mistaken for a need for food or medication. With age the body loses the ability to signal to us its need for water, yet many conditions can be relieved just by drinking this life-giving liquid: back pain, headache, joint pain, heartburn, stomach pain, high blood pressure, cholesterol, excess weight and allergies. Water is essential for the most basic chemical reactions in the body to take place: it activates the enzymes, carries nutrients to the cells and waste matter out of the cells. Our bodies are 60 per cent water so it's hardly surprising that it is so vital.

Dr Batmanghelidj recommends drinking at least 2 litres a day in addition to any other beverages. If you do not feel thirsty it does not mean you do not need water – it means your thirst mechanisms are out of order.

You will also do your body a lot of good by including our Green Tea with Ginger drink in your diet. In one sip you have the beneficial antioxidants of green tea and the digestive properties of the ginger. Read more about the properties of these two plants on pages 161–162.

A glass of red wine a day may help keep your cardiovascular system in good working order. Not just any bottle of red wine, though. French research shows that the older and renowned wines made in the traditional way have more antioxidant activity.

# type a: health issues

**Digestion**

Having good digestion is the first step to good health. For type As to function at their best, they need to take into account their particular digestive characteristics. Type As tend to have low stomach acid (hydrochloric acid) and therefore low digestive enzymes. Eating a meal sets in motion the production of stomach acid that in turn indicates to the digestive system that it should produce digestive enzymes. So if your stomach acid is low your digestive enzymes will also be low. By following the guidance given in the paragraph on protein consumption you will avoid overtaxing your system.

Incomplete digestion leads to toxicity which in turn produces signs of dysfunction that can affect all the systems of the body. Here are just a few symptoms of a toxic body: headaches, eye problems, ear problems, respiratory problems such as excessive mucus formation, frequent need to clear the throat, blood sugar irregularities, muscle/joint aches and pains, skin problems, anxiety and irritability.

Following your blood type diet and avoiding the foods containing the lectins detrimental to your health will maximize digestion and help avoid bloating, flatulence and gripping pains in the stomach.

**Weight**

If you have a weight problem you need to tackle it differently from type O. You should stick to your diet and avoid meat, making sure you get sufficient protein at each meal in the form of fish, poultry, tofu, eggs and beans. Make the right grain choices, avoid wheat and eat very small amounts of dairy produce – one or two yogurts or pieces of cheese per week (sheep's or goat's, not cow's). Eat plenty of vegetables as always. Remember that weight loss has more to do with food choices than calories.

I have found that stress is an important element in weight problems. Consider doing a test that measures the stress hormones produced by the adrenal glands: cortisol and DHEA (dehydroepiandrosterone). I have conducted hundreds of adrenal stress tests with my patients and type As definitely have the highest cortisol levels. If this condition is long-standing the patient may already be in a state of adrenal fatigue, which results in low energy levels and difficulty coping with any type of stress.

High cortisol levels can decrease muscle mass and increase blood sugar levels, both of which lead to weight gain – particularly around the waist. If, as an A, you have difficulty losing weight you might want to look into your stress hormone levels. It doesn't take much for them to skyrocket in your system. Seek out a nutritionist who is familiar with this issue and who can help you with natural substances such as siberian ginseng, vitamin $B_5$, phosphatidylserine, vitamin C and others. They do work very well in restoring adrenal health and assisting fat loss and muscle gain.

---

# Constance

Blood Type A
Age 26

I have always struggled with my weight. Since adolescence I have tried various diets that have worked to some degree but I have never found anything that seemed right for me. I can compare this to a key trying to find the right lock. Sometimes the lock seems to be the right one but it is never the perfect fit. With this way of eating I have finally found the right key. I have learned to listen to what my body has to tell me. With this way of eating (I use this phrase because the word diet has rather restrictive connotations) I have experienced a heightened sense of well-being. I had acne and lots of bloating after meals or in hot weather. After certain meals I would become apathetic and want to sleep. I also had tendonitis in my knees that didn't respond to medical or alternative treatment. After several months of this new way of eating all my problems gradually disappeared.

---

### Heart Disease

Take care of your heart and arteries. In mainstream medicine elevated cholesterol is considered a risk factor for cardiovascular disease. If one looks more closely one realizes that heart disease is not necessarily linked with elevated cholesterol. Studies have shown that not everyone with cardiovascular disease has a high cholesterol level. According to research into blood types and heart disease, blood types A and AB tend to have higher cholesterol levels than Os and Bs. Elevated cholesterol levels therefore seem to be more of a risk factor for heart disease in As and ABs than Os and Bs. Here is another one of those blood type links that could explain the partial success which the official "good for your heart" diet recommendations have in reducing cholesterol levels and heart attacks. These recommendations are close to what type As should be eating, so As will have good results with such diets. One of my patients who is an O was put on a diet of beans, grains and little meat. Her blood cholesterol level jumped from 199 to 233 in less than 2 years. After 5 months of following the blood type diet for type O and eating red meat and hardly any grains or cheese her blood cholesterol dropped from from 233 to 171. The reason I mention this type O patient here is because she was eating a type A diet although she is an O. The diet that enabled her cholesterol levels to drop was the diet appropriate for her blood type and not the generally accepted cholesterol-lowering diet.

Following your blood type A diet will help you reduce your cholesterol levels if they are high. Legumes and lentils, vegetables (artichokes, carrots, beetroot, garlic, onions, leeks), fruits (apples, avocados, grapefruit, pineapple), fatty fish with their beneficial oils (mackerel, sardines, salmon, tuna, herring), soya bean products, brown rice and oats, olive oil, walnuts and almonds – scientific studies have shown that all these foods lower cholesterol levels. Even if your levels are normal, you will benefit from this diet as it will prevent cholesterol levels from rising. You may eat eggs; although they do contain cholesterol they have never been shown to substantially raise cholesterol levels. High levels of cholesterol mainly come from the fact that our body manufactures it from sugar and synthesises it from fats. Some of us are better at this than others, As and ABs for instance.

Another factor in cardiovascular disease is the thickness of your blood. Around 80 per cent of strokes and heart attacks are due to a blood clot. Blood type A has more active blood clotting factors than type O, so As should eat foods that have been shown to help control blood clotting. Garlic is a very important one. Crush raw garlic in your salad dressings and use lemon juice instead of vinegar; the crushing and the acid from the lemon juice help release a substance called ajoene, a very potent anticoagulant. Onions are another amazing food that can neutralize blood clots, while fatty fish contain compounds that have anticlotting properties. And the good news for all wine lovers is that drinking one glass of good quality red wine with your main meal will help prevent blood clotting. Resveratrol – a substance produced by the fermentation of grape skins – has been shown to prevent blood platelets from clumping together. You can also drink red grape juice, but you will need three times as much to get the same benefit as one glass of wine. Another important drink is green tea, which contains a clot-dissolving compound called catechin. Finally, include olive oil and fresh pineapple in your diet as they have been shown to protect the arteries.

If you include all of these foods in your everyday diet you will be giving your body the best chance of long-term good health.

## Cancer

There is a clear association between blood types A and AB and cancer. Certain inherent factors in blood type A make this blood type friendly territory for the development of cancer. When cancer cells develop in As they tend to be accepted by the immune system as friends instead of being fought and killed. Of course there are many other factors that come into play but following the blood type diet can play a powerful part in avoiding cancer.

Apart from the foods that have been shown to be protective against cancer in general and even help prevent the spread of cancer, Dr D'Adamo's research has discovered some foods that are specifically beneficial for blood type A (and AB) in the fight against cancer. Snails – the kind you eat in France in a parsley and garlic sauce – contain a lectin that has anti-cancer properties specially suited to type A (and AB). This lectin has anti-cancer activity towards breast cancer cells. Shelled, unskinned peanuts offer the same benefits. Lentils, the common domestic mushroom and the grain amaranth are also recommended for their anti-cancer effects.

Soya has been shown in many studies to protect against cancer, and is specially well suited for type As (and ABs). Among other foods that are highly recommended are fruits and vegetables. They contain nutrients, phytonutrients and fibre that have been shown to have these protective effects. Eating large amounts of fruits and vegetables can cut your cancer risk in half. The general recommendation is to eat at least 5 portions of fruit and vegetables every day. In this case more is better.

Garlic and onions have been shown in studies to contain substances that prevented laboratory animals from getting cancer – even though they were exposed to potent carcinogens. Green vegetables such as spinach, kale and broccoli are packed with anti-cancer substances that are not destroyed during cooking. Grapefruits and lemons – the whole fruit, including the pith – also have a collection of anti-cancer compounds. One of the best ways of benefiting from all the goodness of these citrus fruits is to add them to your freshly-juiced vegetables. Leave the thin yellow skin on the lemons but remove the coloured skin from the grapefruit. Pineapple is well known as a digestive aid but less well known for its anti-cancer properties. The enzyme bromelain in pineapple appears to activate the immune system to help the body combat cancer cells. Research by Dr Taussig in Hawaii has shown that pineapple inhibits the formation of tumours. Legumes, a beneficial food for type A, also have anti-cancer qualities.

# blood type b: general food recommendations

This blood type, the third to have appeared on earth, is thought to have developed from the earlier blood type O after migrations to the Himalayan regions and later to northern China. The eating habits of these early migrants included meat and fermented milk products. Today, blood type B is the lucky one when it comes to milk products. However, giving you the green light to eat milk products does not mean you can go overboard with full fat cheeses – practise moderation.

In many Asian and African cultures dairy foods have not been part of the diet for generations. If you are a type B who belongs to one of these groups, you may need to introduce dairy products gradually and include a digestive enzyme containing lactase in your diet.

Your body likes meat, fish, dairy products, legumes, nuts and seeds, grains, vegetables and fruits – as long as you choose the right foods in each group. In other words your blood type enables you to eat foods from every category, quite unlike Os and As who are restricted in certain categories. However, there are some meats, fish, legumes and grains that you should avoid.

## Meat, Poultry and Game

Meat is a good food for you and you digest it well. Your best choices are lamb, mutton, rabbit and venison. In our recipes you will find out how to prepare venison – it is the most natural of all meats because these animals live in the wild. You need to avoid chicken as it contains a damaging lectin for your system. You may eat turkey and pheasant (during the hunting season) as well as beef and veal. Your body also has the necessary enzymes to deal with the fats in these foods so do not worry about eating some saturated fat.

## Seafood

Fish is another good source of protein for type B, although some are to be avoided – such as anchovy, sea bass and smoked salmon. Make it a point to eat fatty fish (mackerel, sardines, fresh salmon, tuna, herring) that contain beneficial omega-3 oils. Shellfish is definitely not for you because of the presence of lectins that act against your B makeup.

## Milk Products

When it comes to milk, cheese and yogurt you are the lucky one. You may use dairy products as a source of protein, but if you are prone to respiratory infections or problems with excess mucus formation avoid these foods for some time as they encourage these problems. If your body is not accustomed to dairy products, start slowly. You may need to add the digestive enzyme lactase in capsule form and start with predigested forms of milk products, such as yogurt and kefir.

As you will see in the section on health issues for your type, your immune system needs special care. Research has shown that yogurt can stimulate different aspects of immunity, enabling your system to fight against bacteria and viruses.

---

# Marie

Blood Type B
Age 43

For many years I had been carrying around chronic fatigue like a millstone around my neck, despite eating organic food and taking supplements. For two years premenstrual problems have been plaguing me for 4–5 days each month. Since starting the blood type diet some months ago and changing my supplements, I no longer suffer from pre-menstrual syndrome and my need for daily afternoon naps has almost disappeared.

---

## Legumes

With a few notable exceptions, these are another good source of protein for type Bs. You may eat a portion of legumes nearly every day. They are a source of fibre that encourages good bowel function and helps regulate blood sugar levels. Avoid lentils. In addition, soya beans and soya bean products are not really for you. For various reasons they react negatively with your system. I have noticed many of my B patients naturally avoid them.

## Grains

Grains are a concentrated source of carbohydrate, and type Bs need to watch their consumption of grains and carbohydrates in general. Wheat, corn, buckwheat and rye should be avoided by this blood type. They contain lectins that block insulin activity, thereby disrupting the way sugar is metabolized in the body. Instead of sugar being used for energy it can be stored as fat and cause weight gain. Also, this excess of sugar in the blood can form elevated levels of a type of blood lipids called triglycerides that are also a risk factor for heart disease.

This doesn't bar you from eating all grains. Try spelt instead of wheat. This ancient grain can replace wheat in nearly every circumstance: pies, cakes, breads, pasta etc. Rice and oats are also very good for you. You may eat sprouted grains. The best source is Essene bread (also called sprouted wheat bread). Although it is made with wheat, sprouting destroys the lectins that normally should be avoided. For more information on Essene bread see page 10.

## Nuts, Seeds and their Oils

In our diet we lack one family of oils called omega-3 fatty acids. These are found in walnuts and flaxseeds (linseeds). It is important to regularly incorporate these seeds in your diet. Walnut and flaxseed oils are very prone to rancidity because the omega-3 fatty acids they contain are very fragile and can easily suffer from oxidation. Buy from a reputable manufacturer, keep these oils in the refrigerator and use within six weeks of opening.

There are quite a lot of commonly eaten nuts and seeds that type Bs need to avoid, mainly because of the agglutinating lectins they contain. Avoid peanuts, cashews, pine nuts, pistachios, pumpkin seeds, hazelnuts, sesame seeds and sunflower seeds. Avoid all oils made with these nuts and seeds including canola, soy and corn. You can enjoy walnuts, linseeds, almonds, brazil nuts, pecans and macadamia nuts. The best cooking oil is olive oil and for salads choose flaxseed, walnut and olive oil.

---

## Fats and Oils

Nuts and seeds contain some essential fats, and because these fatty acids are "essential" a deficiency can greatly compromise our health. Up until about 50 years ago nuts and seeds were cold pressed in local mills, where people would regularly buy a fresh supply. Today, refined oils are the norm. These may last a long time in the bottle but they have little of the health-giving qualities of cold pressed oils and can have a detrimental effect on health.

It would take many, many pages to write about all the health benefits of fats and oils. Suffice it to say that every cell in the body, in order to function properly, needs the right fatty acids. And given that our cells are what make up our tissues, our organs and ultimately our bodies, should we not be giving them the best possible sustenance? If at all possible avoid industry-made oils and use the best quality cold pressed oils you can find – buy from a reputable manufacturer, keep the oil in the refrigerator and use within six weeks of opening. France is walnut country and cold pressed walnut oil can be easily found. I regularly recommend eating walnuts and using walnut oil in salads. Many people use olive oil in salads but it does not contain essential fatty acids.

---

## Vegetables

All blood groups benefit from eating plenty of vegetables. Along with fruits, they are the basis of a healthy diet. Ensure they are as fresh as possible and eat them every day for lunch and dinner – raw or cooked, juiced, in salads, in soup – and as a snack. In the recipe section you will read about the tremendous benefits of eating these health-giving plants.

Green leafy vegetables such as kale, spring cabbage, spring greens (collards), turnip greens and dandelion leaves should be a regular part of your diet as they contain high levels of carotenoids and magnesium. Avoid tomatoes as they contain a lectin that is detrimental to the type B system. Corn should also be avoided.

Magnesium is a mineral you should be regularly obtaining through your diet. It is needed in high amounts in times of stress. Milk and cheese both contain magnesium, as well as calcium. Kale, however, contains about the same amount of calcium as milk but three times as much magnesium – yet another reason not to overlook those green leafy vegetables.

As a type B your immune system can be your weak point. Protect yourself against bacterial and viral infections by eating large helpings of vegetables. Garlic, maitake and shiitake mushrooms have been shown to boost immunity and you can also find them in capsule form.

## Fruits

You may eat just about all fruits available. Vegetables and fruits are similar in their nutrient content and are our best source of vitamins, minerals, phytonutrients and antioxidants. Fruits generally have less minerals and a higher sugar content than vegetables. However, the sugar comes in the form of fructose, which raises blood sugar levels much less rapidly than sucrose – the sugar found in table sugar and refined carbohydrates such as white flour. This is an important difference. Fruit can help maintain balanced energy levels, while refined sugars can make them fluctuate wildly.

If you wish to lose weight eat a piece of fruit 30 minutes before your meals. This practice has been shown to moderate appetite and encourage weight loss. However, if you eat fruit as a mid-morning or mid-afternoon snack it is wise to eat some form of protein with it in order to maintain good blood sugar levels. You could have a yogurt, a piece of cheese, or some walnuts. Balancing protein and carbohydrates helps ensure more even blood sugar levels.

# Seham

Blood Type B
Age 37

---

The blood type diet has improved a number of health aspects that had been irritating me for years. I now have much better digestion and feel light rather than bloated after meals. I have less fatigue and my energy levels are more constant throughout the day. This diet has also helped me lose some weight. Another slight but nonetheless irritating problem was that I used to spend a good part of the morning blowing my nose. Thankfully I am now rid of my nasal congestion and runny nose.

---

### What Can I Drink?

Green tea should be your number one choice. Apart from the cancer and cardio-vascular protective benefits ascribed to it on page 162, green tea also has immune-stimulating effects that are particularly relevant for the sensitive B immune system. Green tea polyphenols, the active ingredient, have been shown to act in two ways to protect against micro-organisms: they enhance the body's defence mechanisms and act on the micro-organisms themselves, making them less potent. See the food list on page 45 for other suitable drinks for type Bs.

## type b: health issues

### Weight and Sugar Metabolism

If you have a weight problem it may be enough for you simply to follow your blood type diet, as the lectins in certain foods can disrupt the way your body deals with sugar. These lectins can have an insulin-like effect on the cells. If the cells are continuously stimulated in this way they will transform sugar into fat and store it, instead of burning it as fuel. Too much insulin-like stimulation creates a condition called insulin resistance in which the cells no longer respond to insulin as they should. Dr D'Adamo has found that the lectins in wheat, corn, buckwheat, lentils, sesame seeds and peanuts have a detrimental effect on blood sugar metabolism in blood type B.

Another strategy that is helpful for type Bs is eating enough protein to balance out your carbohydrate intake. This will enable the two hormones that regulate blood sugar levels – insulin and glucagon – to work in harmony.

Some people are very sensitive to the protein/carbohydrate ratio and would benefit from ensuring this ratio is balanced at every meal and snack. For breakfast you may start out by replacing bread and the usual jam with bread and cheese or bread with a scrambled egg. For lunch and dinner always eat one of your good sources of protein with plenty of vegetables and some grains. Here is a visual tip to help balance protein and carbohydrates. Fill one quarter of the surface of your plate with protein (meat, fish, fowl or eggs) and the rest with mainly vegetables and a little rice or other grain. If you eat legumes at a meal, avoid grains as legumes are half protein and half carbohydrate. I find this way of balancing a meal is useful in helping my patients to balance their blood sugar levels and promote insulin efficiency.

# Michel

Blood Type B
Age 54

It is not possible for me to state categorically that my good health and controlled weight are essentially due to the blood type diet; to my general care about what I eat and how, to the few nutrients that complement my diet, or to my good nature. Yet despite long work days, nights that are often too short and a fair amount of urban stress, I feel better than ever and now get through the winter without the usual cold.

What I can say with certainty is that (at least to me, a type B) following the blood type diet has neither become constraining, inconvenient nor cumbersome. I just choose the right thing when I have the choice. Every time I have no better choice at hand, or from time to time when I just feel strongly like it, I derogate without guilt. My guidelines are to be cautious about the foods that form the basis of my diet. Thus no one needs to notice and I don't feel constrained either. I should even add that the blood type diet makes a quite lively and interesting topic for discussion around the dining table.

## Your Immune System needs Support

I have found some of the most resistant bacterial infections in my B patients. As a precaution against any micro-organisms taking hold in your body eat plenty of the foods that have been shown to boost immunity. Vegetables and fruits in general are great for this, as is green tea (see page 161). Garlic is especially good, so add it to your salad dressing every day. Onions have potent antibacterial and antiviral activity – Russian scientists have extensively studied this effect. Chilli peppers, cayenne pepper and horseradish have also been shown to help with infections. And don't forget, you are in the lucky group that is able to eat yogurt with its immune-stimulating power.

You should also ensure you consume a reasonable amount of fat in your diet and, above all, that you get the right ones. Eat fatty fish such as mackerel, sardines, tuna and salmon; and use flaxseed oil and walnut oil in your salads. They will all provide beneficial omega-3 oils.

# blood type ab: general food recommendations

Unlike the other blood types, AB was not part of the evolutionary process but is the result of the mixing of types A and B. Type AB has been around for only about 1,000 years and makes up a mere five per cent of the population of the planet.

The French psychologist, Leone Bourdel, once described type AB as "the richest of the four temperaments as it possesses the advantages of the other three, but it is also the victim of its incompatibilities and is made of contradictions and incoherence". In terms of food choices this same pattern shows up. Type AB is complex, sometimes resembling an A, sometimes a B and at other times it resembles its far away blood type ancestor type O.

I have noticed that several of my type AB patients have, on their own, adopted some eating habits that tie in with the findings of the research into blood type eating. They tend to have smaller meals which are easier to digest, they eat meat in reduced quantities, enjoy a good breakfast that includes some form of protein, and stick to regular mealtimes. All these steps ensure type ABs feel better and have more energy.

## Meat and Poultry

With regard to digesting meat you resemble type A – your stomach acid tends to be low and digestive enzymes are lacking. Limit yourself to occasionally eating lamb, turkey and rabbit. When it comes to chicken, duck and guinea fowl you resemble type B and should avoid them.

## Seafood

If you are not used to eating fish, increasing your intake of this valuable source of protein will significantly improve your diet. The A in you may make you prone to high cholesterol levels and eating fish rich in omega-3 fatty acids will help prevent and reduce this cardiovascular risk factor. The best fish for you are mackerel, sardines, tuna, herring and salmon (wild if possible). You can also eat fish that are not rich in fatty acids, as these contain other elements that benefit the cardiovascular system. You may eat mussels and scallops but avoid other shellfish.

## Soya Products and Legumes

Tofu and tempeh are easily digestible protein sources for you. Legumes and lentils can be enjoyed almost every day, although you must stick to the ones without detrimental lectins. Lentils, broad (fava) beans, cannellini beans, white beans, pinto and northern beans are on your list. They provide a good source of complex carbohydrates and fibre. Legumes contain phytosterols and fibre that have cholesterol-lowering and cancer-protective effects. In addition, legumes encourage good bowel function, which protects against colon cancer and haemorrhoids.

Soya beans and the other legumes have approximately the same qualities. However, soya beans, and hence soya products, have a higher fat content, plenty of

essential fatty acids, a higher protein content and an excellent amino acid profile.
Soya is a good source of lecithin, which has been shown to lower cholesterol levels and help the liver and gall bladder do their work.

Soya also contains phytoestrogens that exert both a mild estrogenic and anti-estrogenic effect. In other words these compounds have a balancing effect on the hormonal system.

## Grains

Cereals, breads and pasta are all made with grains. Type AB have adapted to this food category and you should therefore be able to enjoy them in your daily fare. Just make sure your consumption doesn't push out the vegetables from your diet. As with all blood types, wheat is to be avoided if you have a weight problem and easy build-up of mucus in the respiratory tract. Vary your grain choices: eat millet, oats, rye, spelt, quinoa, rice and wheat if you can in view of the above considerations. Avoid corn and buckwheat.

If you have blood sugar irregularities in association with weight gain you will need to limit your grain consumption. You may eat sprouted grains as found in Essene bread (also called sprouted wheat bread). Although this is made with wheat, the sprouting process destroys the lectins that should normally be avoided. For more information on Essene bread see page 10.

## Milk Products

This is where your B aspect comes into play. You can eat cheeses made from cow's, sheep's or goat's milk, as well as yogurt and kefir. However, be aware of the fact that cheese does contain saturated fat and that your body could make excessive amounts of cholesterol from this fat. Milk products can also encourage mucus production in susceptible people. If you regularly develop respiratory problems or have a chronic condition such as asthma or hay fever, you may benefit from avoiding milk products for several months. Reintroduce them gradually once your immune system has become stronger.

## Nuts, Seeds and their Oils

Nuts and seeds are a source of protein and fibre. Some contain valuable essential fatty acids and should be included regularly in the diet: walnuts and flaxseeds (linseeds) are my favourites and both are suitable for ABs.

The essential fatty acids in walnuts and flaxseeds are effective in reducing cholesterol levels and are a valuable food for good brain function. Walnuts and flaxseeds have a very cleansing effect in the intestinal tract, the seat of a great part of our immune system. Flaxseeds contain lignans that are transformed in the gut into substances that have anti-cancer effects. In the following section on health issues for ABs you will see that you need to be especially careful to protect yourself against cancer. Flaxseeds also reduce cholesterol levels. The omega-3 oils in walnuts and flaxseeds are beneficial for inflammatory and allergic conditions such as asthma and eczema.

Eat walnuts and flaxseeds regularly. In order to benefit from the essential fatty acids in flaxseeds it is important to reduce them to a powder before eating them. Grind them in an electric coffee grinder, keep in a refrigerator for no longer than five days and sprinkle 1–3 tablespoons on your food or mix in a glass of water and drink. Flaxseeds work wonders against constipation.

---

# Afsaneh

Blood Type AB
Age 45

I suffered for many years from bloating, migraine, terrible nausea and constant fatigue. I was also overweight, and decided to turn to a nutritionist for help. On her advice, I began following the blood type diet and took appropriate herbs and nutrients for my condition.

In the beginning I found it difficult. At one point I was even quite discouraged as the initial results were poor. But I must admit I wasn't following the recommendations very well. I set my mind on doing it seriously and felt the results within days. I had no more headaches or nausea and I lost weight.

Then I went on a two-week holiday to visit my family in an area of France where the staple foods are potatoes, pork, plenty of home-made cakes, wine and alcohol. I could not follow the blood type diet correctly but I tried my best. I ate as many vegetables and salads as possible and bought my own rye bread. I didn't get the usual head-cracking migraines and was less constipated. Although certain symptoms came back, I still saw the benefits in the fact that my addiction for coffee had stopped and all the things that I used to like (coke, fried foods and white bread) didn't appeal to me at all. After previous weight-loss diets, I would have cravings for chocolate, sugar and rich, creamy foods but for the first time my body wanted what was best for it.

---

## Vegetables

Eat vegetables as often as you can. In our modern civilisation we have a tendency to eat too few vegetables for various reasons: they take some time to prepare (but really not that much), you need to shop more often because they need to be fresh, and many adults and children claim they do not like them.

Vegetables are the basis of a healthy diet. Ensure they are as fresh as possible and eat them every day for lunch and dinner – raw or cooked, juiced, in salads, in soup – and as a snack. You will find information about the tremendous benefits of eating these health-giving plants in the recipe section. Make green leafy vegetables such as kale, spring greens (collards), turnip greens and dandelion leaves a regular part of your diet as they contain high levels of carotenoids and magnesium.

Magnesium is a mineral you should be regularly obtaining through your diet. It is needed in high amounts in times of stress. Milk and cheese both contain magnesium, as well as calcium. Kale, however, contains about the same amount of calcium as milk but three times as much magnesium – yet another reason not to overlook those green leafy vegetables.

When making salad dressing avoid vinegar, which may irritate your stomach, and replace it with lemon juice. Use plenty of fresh herbs and regularly add garlic, which has anti-cancer, antimicrobial and cardiovascular effects. For your salad dressings use cold pressed walnut or flaxseed oil. For cooking, the only oil that will withstand the heat is olive oil. Do not heat cold pressed oils.

## Fruit

Fruits are rich in phytonutrients and vitamins. Some of the fruits commonly eaten have been studied and are shown to have anti-cancer, anti-inflammatory, antibacterial and antiviral effects. Blueberries and blackcurrants contain phytonutrients called anthocyanosides that strengthen blood vessel walls, protecting against arterial damage that can lead to cardiovascular disease. Apricots are rich in beta carotene and therefore protective against cancer. The Japanese have also isolated an anti-cancer substance in figs. Grapefruit (and other citrus fruits) have been shown to reduce the risk of cancer, and to lower cholesterol. For this latter effect you must go for the whole fruit and not just the juice. Strawberries reduce cholesterol and can block nitrosamines, a potent cancer-causing compound.

All these fruits and more are yours to eat and will contribute to your protection against cancer and cardiovascular disease – some health aspects you must particularly protect yourself from.

## What Can I Drink?

Green tea is your best choice. It has cancer and cardiovascular protective benefits. Many Japanese studies have shown that drinking green tea (about 10 cups a day) reduces cholesterol levels, prevents the formation of blood clots and also helps relax blood vessel walls thus reducing high blood pressure. For other drinks see the food list on page 47.

# type ab: health issues

## Digestion

Your digestive makeup when it comes to protein resembles that of blood type A and blood type B. This means that you can eat a bit more animal protein than blood type A but should still watch the quantities at each sitting. You do not have enough stomach acid to digest large quantities of meat at a time. Overtaxing your system with foods that are not going to be properly metabolized will create toxicity in the digestive tract and then in the general system. This can cause symptoms such as headaches, eye problems, ear problems, respiratory problems such as excessive mucus formation, frequent need to clear the throat, blood sugar irregularities, muscle/joint aches and pains, skin problems, anxiety and irritability – to name but a few. Toxicity is also a forerunner of cancer, a health issue type ABs need to look out for.

Faulty digestion linked with too much animal protein and also the wrong choices can be a factor in weight gain.

## Weight

Your weight has less to do with the amount of calories eaten than with what happens with sugar (glucose) and fats that enter your body – in other words your metabolism. Metabolism is the chemical and physical reactions that take place in our cells to turn fat and sugar into energy and protein into cells. The rate at which this happens varies from one person to the next. Some people have a slow metabolism and will put on weight easily. Others have a fast metabolism and will not put on weight even if they eat a lot. The efficiency with which you burn carbohydrates and fats to produce energy rather than to stock them in fat cells, will determine your capacity to lose weight and to remain slim. Lectins, exercise and specific nutrients involved in energy production all have their role to play here.

The lectins you should avoid can slow down your metabolism. They can block the proper utilization of insulin by the cells and cause insulin resistance. This means that despite the production of insulin your cells do not respond to it as they should and if this goes on for a long time the pancreas ends up producing more and more insulin that is actually not doing its job. The consequence of all this is that the sugar needed by the cells to produce energy is actually driven in another direction to be stored as body fat – and the upward scale to weight gain has begun. In many of my patients I have noticed that just by making the proper food choices (avoiding the bad lectins), without specially avoiding the foods that are traditionally thought of as being "fattening", the pounds start falling off.

As with the other blood groups your best move is to stop eating the foods containing the lectins you should avoid, as well as those that are not going to be properly digested. Although most ABs who are in a state of good health should be able to eat wheat, if you need to lose weight avoid this grain. Refrain from eating large quantities of animal protein at each meal because you will have problems digesting it completely and therefore accumulate toxins. Remember the A in you restricts the amount of meat you should be eating. Instead choose tofu, tempeh, fish and milk products from your list of acceptable foods, as these are good muscle-building protein sources for you. You need to have a good active muscle mass in order to facilitate the chemical reactions that are going to enable you to burn fat to make energy.

## Heart Disease

When it comes to cardiovascular health, you express the A in you. Take care of your cholesterol levels, check your blood pressure, reduce your stress and eat the foods that will keep you from forming blood clots.

Following the blood type diet will help you reduce your cholesterol levels if they are high, so choose legumes and lentils, tofu and tempeh, vegetables (carrots, garlic, onions, leeks), fruits (apples, grapefruit, pineapple), fatty fish with their beneficial oils (mackerel, sardines, salmon, tuna, herring), soya bean products, brown rice and oats, olive oil, walnuts and almonds. All these foods have been shown in scientific studies to lower cholesterol levels. Even if your levels are normal, you will benefit from this diet as it will prevent cholesterol levels from rising. You may eat eggs, although they do contain cholesterol. Eating eggs has never been shown to substantially raise cholesterol levels, so do not deprive yourself of this excellent food. High levels of cholesterol mainly come from the fact that our body manufactures it from sugar and synthesises it from fats. Some of us are better at this than others, As and ABs for instance.

You may continue to eat some meat as long as you stick to approximately three servings per week. Eat brazil nuts as they contain a surprising amount of selenium – between 200 and 5,000mcg of selenium per 100 grams. Selenium has been shown to help prevent oxidation of cholesterol and prevent platelet aggregation, a possible factor in blood clots. A Finnish study has shown that the more selenium you have in your blood the less likely you are to die of a heart attack. Other good sources of selenium are tuna, swordfish, liver and garlic.

Another aspect in cardiovascular disease is the thickness of your blood. Around 80 per cent of strokes and heart attacks are due to a blood clot. Your best bet is to eat the foods that have been shown to help control blood clotting. Garlic is a very important one. Crush raw garlic in your salad dressings and use lemon juice instead of vinegar; the crushing and the acid from the lemon juice help release a substance called ajoene, a very potent anticoagulant. Onions are another amazing food that can neutralize blood clots that could form after eating a meal high in fats. Fatty fish are also valuable: the oils, as well as other compounds in fish, have anti-clotting activity. Drinking one glass of good quality red wine with your main meal will help prevent blood clotting. Resveratrol is a substance produced by the fermentation of grape skins during the making of red wine; it has been shown to prevent blood platelets from clumping together. You can also drink red grape juice, but you will need three times as much to get the same benefit as one glass of wine. Green tea contains a clot-dissolving compound called catechin. Including olive oil in your diet is another golden opportunity to protect your arteries against blood clots. Fresh pineapple has also been shown to protect the arteries.

## Patricia

Blood Type AB
Age 42

Since adolescence I have been struggling with my diet. Today I am a violin soloist and at 14 years of age I began my first exams. My mother forced me to eat meat because she thought it would give me extra strength. I invariably noticed that my digestion would be sluggish and heavy and that I wanted to sleep after meals. I also had severe stomach burning after breakfasts consisting of orange juice, bread and black tea.

For 20 years I went from one diet to another, losing weight then gaining more than I had lost. Digestion was always a problem. My life as a solo musician was very demanding so my stress levels were high. At age 38, I divorced and went into a depression that lasted nine months. Another episode of dieting made me lose 20kg and gain 25.

When I first saw Karen I had an underfunctioning thyroid and my attitude to food was one of disgust. By following the blood type diet I rediscovered the foods that I liked as a child and was naturally inclined to eat. After three months my digestion became normal again – no more stomach burn and bloating. My vitality has returned and I have good positive energy for performing. My leg cramps are almost gone and my skin allergies have disappeared. I don't feel the irrepressible need for sugar and my cravings have disappeared, the oedema in my ankles has gone and my memory has improved. Today I take pleasure in eating the foods that are good for my blood type because it is actually the food that I like. I also remain wide awake after meals!

## Cancer

There is a clear association between blood types A and AB and cancer. This does not mean that you will get cancer, nor does it mean that blood type O and B will not get cancer. It means that being an A or an AB is another risk factor such as smoking, being in contact with environmental carcinogens, having nutrient deficiencies, eating a bad diet etc … Certain inherent factors in blood type AB make this blood type a friendly ground for the development of cancer. When cancer cells develop in ABs they tend to be accepted by the immune system as friends instead of being fought and killed.

However, with all we know now about cancer prevention – the value of stress reduction, hormone balance (estrogen/progesterone), research into foods, nutrients with anti-cancer activity and now more recently with the blood type diets – it is possible to take various steps to prevent its development.

Apart from the foods that have been shown to be protective against cancer in general and even help avoid the spread of cancer, Dr D'Adamo in his research has discovered that some foods are specifically beneficial for blood type AB in the fight against cancer. Snails – the kind you eat in France in a parsley and garlic sauce – contain a lectin that has anti-cancer properties specially suited to type AB. Peanuts (in their red skins), a beneficial food for ABs, also have a lectin with anti-cancer activity towards breast cancer cells and cancer cells in general. Lentils and the grain amaranth are also recommended for their anti-cancer effects.

Soya, which has been shown extensively in studies to protect against cancer, is especially well suited to ABs. Among the other foods that are highly recommended are fruits and vegetables. They contain nutrients, phytonutrients and fibre that have all been shown to have these protective effects. Eating large amounts of fruits and vegetables can do as much as cut your cancer risk in half. According to the American National Cancer Institute, you should be eating at least five portions of fruit and vegetables every day. In this case more is better.

Garlic and onions have been shown in studies to contain substances that prevented laboratory animals from getting cancer – even though they were exposed to potent carcinogens. Green vegetables such as spinach, kale and broccoli are packed with anti-cancer substances that are not destroyed during cooking. Most of the cancer-protective nutrients are in the dark green leaves so do not discard these from vegetables such as cabbage. Grapefruits and lemons – the whole fruit, including the pith – also have a collection of anti-cancer compounds. One of the best ways of benefiting from all the goodness of these citrus fruits is to add them to your freshly-juiced vegetables. You may leave the thin yellow skin on the lemons but remove the coloured skin from the grapefruit.

Pineapple is well known as a digestive aid but less well known for its anti-cancer properties. The enzyme bromelain in pineapple appears to activate the immune system to help the body combat cancer cells. Research by Dr Taussig in Hawaii has shown that pineapple inhibits the formation of tumours. Brussels sprouts and broccoli contain indoles that can protect against cancer, especially breast cancer. Legumes, a beneficial food for type AB, also have anti-cancer qualities.

# a final word

The intention with this book is to get you started on the blood type diet so that you can discover its benefits for yourself. I encourage my patients to follow the recommendations for one month and then to re-evaluate. There is nothing like one's own experience for evaluating its effect. But don't be picky about which bits you follow. Do it completely, wholeheartedly. You have nothing to lose. On the contrary, you have much to gain.

Once you have experienced the benefits of "eating right for your type", your body will know what it wants. Some foods that you didn't like at all and that are good for your blood type will begin to seem all right – maybe even very good. This is what I, and my patients, have experienced. However, this does not happen immediately – you must go far enough into the diet to achieve a sense of well-being. I believe that as your body gets healthier it recognizes what it truly needs and your food choices for your blood type become natural. Do be aware, though, that a strong attraction to a food rarely means there is something in it that your body needs. This phenomena often has to do with dependency. For example, sugar cravings recede as you eliminate lectins that have an effect on sugar balance, highly sweet foods, foods you have an intolerance to and when you add certain nutrients. Simply give your body time to reach its natural equilibrium on the blood type diet. Then listen – you will find your body knows what it needs.

# the food lists

The following food lists, though somewhat simplified, are based on the original lists developed by Dr Peter D'Adamo. They are designed to help you make day-to-day decisions about what to include in your diet. If you wish for a more in-depth examination than is possible here, please refer to *Eat Right For Your Type* and *Live Right For Your Type* (see bibliography).

There is one aspect of the blood type diet that we have not addressed here and that is your secretor status. Eighty per cent of the population are secretors and 20 per cent are non-secretors. Secretors secrete their blood type information in their body fluids, while non-secretors do not. As your blood type antigen is your first line of defence, this means that non-secretors have less protection against certain infections (bacterial, fungal), auto-immune diseases and inflammation. The following food lists are for secretors. If you find the diet helps you but not as much as you would like, you may just be a non-secretor. A test will enable you to discover your secretor status (see the resources section). If you are a non-secretor, the status of some foods changes. If you wish to refine your diet to this degree, refer to *Live Right For Your Type*, which studies this issue in detail.

# BLOOD TYPE O

| Food Group | Foods to eat | Foods to avoid | Comments |
|---|---|---|---|
| Meat and poultry | All meat except … All poultry except … | Pork/bacon/ham Quail | Meat is your best source of protein – be sure to regularly eat red meat. Among your best choices of meat are beef, lamb, calves' liver, veal and venison |
| Seafood and snails | All fish except … | Barracuda, catfish, muskellunge, octopus, pollack, squid | Fish, particularly cod, bass, halibut, rainbow trout, snapper, sole and swordfish, are a good source of protein but don't be tempted to eat fish instead of meat – include both in your diet |
| | All shellfish except … Snails | Abalone, conch | |
| Dairy | Butter, clarified butter, goat's cheese, sheep's cheese, mozzarella, goat's and sheep's yogurt | All other cow's milk cheeses, cow's and goat's milk, cow's yogurt | Although you can eat those listed in the first column, limit your consumption to no more than two yogurts and two pieces of cheese per week. Some Os do not tolerate any milk products at all |
| Eggs | Duck egg, chicken egg | Goose egg, quail egg | Up to six a week |
| Oils | Flaxseed/linseed oil, olive oil, canola oil, sesame oil, walnut | Coconut, corn, cottonseed, peanut, safflower, soy, sunflower, wheat germ | Use olive oil for cooking and salads, all others for salads only. Use cider vinegar or lemon juice in dressings |
| Nuts and seeds | Almond, flaxseed/linseed, hazelnut, macadamia, pecan, pine nut, walnut (black, English), pumpkin seeds, sesame seeds | Brazil nut, cashew, chestnut, peanut, pistachio, sunflower seeds, poppy seeds | Include regularly in your eating habits, especially walnuts and ground flaxseeds |
| Legumes and soya products | All beans except … Soya (bean, cheese, milk, miso, tempeh, tofu etc.) | Kidney, lentils (domestic, green, red), haricot (navy), pinto, tamarind | You can eat some beans and soya products but your best sources of protein are meat, poultry and fish. Get your fibre from vegetables |

| Food Group | Foods to eat | Foods to avoid | Comments |
|---|---|---|---|
| Grains | Essene bread (100% sprouted grain bread), buckwheat, kamut, millet, oats, quinoa, rice, rye, spelt, tapioca, wild rice | Barley, corn, sorghum, wheat | Essene bread is made with 100% sprouted grains and is by far the best form of bread for you |
| Vegetables | All except ... | Alfalfa sprouts, capers, cauliflower, cucumber, leek, mushroom (shiitake, domestic), olive (black), pickle, potato (sweet potatoes are OK) | Make vegetables "king" at your table. Eat onions as an actual vegetable |
| Fruits | All except ... | Asian pear, avocado, bitter melon, blackberry, cantaloupe, coconut, honeydew, kiwi, orange, plantain, tangerine | Eat plenty of berries in season. Eat about 450g/1lb of fruit per day |
| Spices | All except ... | Mace, nutmeg, pepper (preground black/white) | Turmeric and ginger are especially suitable due to their anti-inflammatory and digestive qualities |
| Culinary herbs | All | | Parsley is very good for Os so eat it in large quantities and include flat-leaf parsley regularly in your salads |
| Beverages | Green tea, soda water, red wine | Coffee, lager, spirits, tea (black), white wine | |

# BLOOD TYPE A

| Food Group | Foods to eat | Foods to avoid | Comments |
|---|---|---|---|
| Meat and poultry | Chicken, cornish hens, grouse, guinea fowl, ostrich, squab, turkey | Beef, duck, goose, heart, lamb, liver, mutton, partridge, pheasant, pork/bacon/ham, quail, rabbit, veal, venison | Acceptable forms of meat and poultry should be eaten in moderation |
| Seafood and snails | All fish except … | Anchovy, barracuda, bass (bluegill, striped), beluga, bluefish, catfish, caviar, eel, flounder, grouper, haddock, hake, halibut, herring (and kippers), plaice, smoked salmon, octopus, scup, shad, sole, squid, tilefish | Your best choices of fish include cod, mackerel, monkfish, pollack, red snapper, salmon, sardine, trout (rainbow and sea), whiting |
|  | Shellfish: abalone Snails | Avoid all the rest | Snails are a super health food for you |
| Dairy | Feta cheese (from goat's or sheep's milk), clarified butter, goat's cheese, kefir, goat's milk, mozzarella, paneer, ricotta, sheep's cheese, sour cream (low/non fat), yogurt | Butter, buttermilk, cow's milk (skimmed, semi, whole), all other cow's milk cheeses, whey | Although you can eat those dairy products listed in the first column, none are especially beneficial for you – eat at most three yogurts and three pieces of cheese from this list per week. Some may not tolerate milk products at all |
| Eggs | Duck, chicken, goose, quail |  | Up to three per week |
| Oils | Flaxseed/linseed oil, olive oil, walnut oil, canola oil, safflower oil, sesame oil, sunflower oil, wheat germ oil | Coconut oil, corn oil, cottonseed oil, peanut oil | Use olive oil for cooking and salads, all others for salads only. Avoid all types of vinegar in salad dressings, use lemon juice instead |
| Nuts and seeds | All except … | Brazil nut, cashew, pistachio | Include regularly in your eating habits, especially peanuts, walnuts and ground flaxseeds |

| Food Group | Foods to eat | Foods to avoid | Comments |
|------------|--------------|----------------|----------|
| Legumes and soya products | All beans except … <br><br> Soya (bean, cheese, milk, miso, tofu, tempeh etc.) | Chick peas (garbanzos), kidney bean, lima bean, haricot (navy) bean, red bean | Beans and soya bean products in general are an excellent source of protein for you |
| Grains and related products | All except … | Wheat bran, wheat germ | In certain circumstances wheat should be avoided such as in weight problems, inflammation. In any case vary your grains; avoid over-eating wheat |
| Vegetables | All except … | Aubergine (eggplant), cabbage (Chinese, red, white), capers, cassava, chillies, shiitake mushrooms, olive (black, Greek, Spanish), peppers (green, red, yellow), potato, rhubarb, sweet potato, tomato, yam | Make vegetables "king" at your table |
| Fruits | All except … | Banana, coconut, honeydew melon, mango, orange, papaya, plantain, tangerine | Eat about 450g/1lb fruit per day |
| Spices | All except … | Cayenne pepper, chilli powder, pepper (black, white, red) | Turmeric and ginger are especially good due to their anti-inflammatory and digestive properties |
| Culinary herbs | All | | Parsley is very good for As so eat it in large quantities and include flat-leaf parsley regularly in your salads |
| Beverages | Cider, coffee, green tea, wine (red, white) | Fizzy drinks, lager, soda water, spirits, tea (black) | Limit yourself to one cup of coffee a day. Green tea should be your number one choice, and choose red wine over white |

# BLOOD TYPE B

| Food Group | Foods to eat | Foods to avoid | Comments |
|---|---|---|---|
| Meat and poultry | Beef, lamb, calves' liver, mutton, ostrich, pheasant, rabbit, turkey, venison, veal | Chicken, cornish hens, duck, guinea fowl, heart, goose, partridge, pork/bacon/ham, quail, squab | You are also a meat eater like blood type O, but your choice is more restricted. The meats most beneficial to you are lamb, mutton, rabbit and venison |
| Seafood and snails | All fish except … <br><br> Shellfish: scallops | Anchovy, barracuda, bass (bluegill, sea, striped), beluga, butterfish, eel, octopus, pollack, salmon roe <br> Clam, conch, crab, lobster, molluscs, mussels, oyster, shrimp <br> Snail | Very good source of protein – your best choices include cod, flounder, haddock, halibut, mackerel, salmon, shad, sole, sturgeon |
| Dairy | All except … | Blue cheese | The majority of Bs can eat dairy produce and it is a good source of protein. Your best choices include goat's cheese, goat's milk, mozzarella, cottage cheese, feta cheese, cow's milk, yogurt |
| Eggs | Chicken egg | Duck egg, goose egg, quail egg | |
| Oils | Flaxseed/linseed oil, olive oil, walnut oil, wheat germ oil | All others | Use olive oil for salads and cooking, all others for salads only |
| Nuts and seeds | Almond, brazil nut, chestnut, flaxseed/linseed, macadamia, pecan, walnut (black, English) | Cashew, hazelnut, peanut, pine nut, pistachio, poppy seeds, pumpkin seeds, safflower seeds, sesame seeds, sunflower seeds | Include regularly in your diet, especially walnuts and ground flaxseeds |

| Food Group | Foods to eat | Foods to avoid | Comments |
|---|---|---|---|
| Legumes and soya products | Broad (fava) bean, cannellini bean, kidney bean, lima bean, haricot (navy) bean, northern bean, red bean, green bean, white bean, soya bean | Aduki bean, black bean, black-eyed pea, chick peas (garbanzos), lentil (domestic, red, green), mung bean sprouts, pinto bean, tamarind, soya products (cheese, flakes, granules, milk, miso, tempeh) | Another good source of protein. Haricot (navy) beans, kidney beans, and lima beans are your most beneficial choices |
| Grains and related products | Essene bread (100% sprouted grain bread), barley, millet, oats, quinoa, rice, spelt, wheat (semolina, white flour products) | Amaranth, buckwheat/ kasha, corn, kamut, tapioca, rye, sorghum, tapioca, wheat (bran, couscous, germ, gluten flour products, whole wheat products), wild rice | As strange as it may seem refined wheat is better for you than whole wheat. Eat grains in reasonable quantities |
| Vegetables | All except … | Artichoke (domestic, globe, Jerusalem), olives (black, green, Greek, Spanish), pumpkin, radish, rhubarb, tomato | Make vegetables the "king" at your table |
| Fruits | All except … | Avocado, bitter melon, coconut, persimmon, pomegranate, prickly pear, starfruit | Eat about 450g/1lb of fruit per day |
| Spices | All except … | Allspice, cinnamon, pepper (preground black and white) | Make special use of ginger and turmeric for their anti-inflammatory and digestive effects |
| Culinary herbs | All | | Parsley is very good for Bs so eat it in large quantities and include flat-leaf parsley regularly in your salads |
| Beverages | Cider, lager, coffee, tea (green, black), wine (red, white) | Spirits, soda water, fizzy drinks | Green tea should be your beverage of choice |

# BLOOD TYPE AB

| Food Group | Foods to eat | Foods to avoid | Comments |
|---|---|---|---|
| Meat and poultry | Lamb, calves' liver, mutton, ostrich, pheasant, rabbit, turkey | Beef, chicken, cornish hens, duck, goose, grouse, guinea fowl, heart, pork/bacon/ham, partridge, quail, squab, sweetbreads, veal, venison | Eat small quantities of meat |
| Seafood and snails | All fish except … | Anchovy, barracuda, bass (all types), beluga, eel, flounder, haddock, hake, halibut, octopus, salmon roe, sole, trout (brook, rainbow, sea), whiting, yellowtail | An excellent source of protein – your best choices include cod, mackerel, monkfish, pike, red snapper, salmon, sardine, shad, sturgeon, tuna |
| | Shellfish: abalone, mussels, scallops | Clam, conch, crab, lobster, oyster, shrimp | |
| | Snails | | Snails are a super health food for you |
| Dairy | All (including sheep's and goat's products) except … | Blue cheese, brie, butter, buttermilk, camembert, half-and-half, cow's milk (whole), parmesan cheese, provolone cheese | Should be well tolerated in reasonable amounts. Cultured milk products such as yogurt are particularly suitable, as are cottage cheese, feta cheese and goat's milk |
| Eggs | Chicken egg, goose egg, quail egg | Duck egg | |
| Oils | Olive oil, canola oil, flaxseed/linseed oil, peanut oil, soy oil, walnut oil, wheat germ oil | Coconut oil, corn oil, cottonseed oil, safflower oil, sesame oil, sunflower oil | Use olive oil for salads and cooking, all others for salads only. Avoid vinegar in dressings, use lemon juice |
| Nuts and seeds | Almond, brazil nut, cashew, chestnut, flaxseed/linseed, macadamia, peanut, pecan, pine nut, pistachio, walnut (English, black) | Hazelnut, poppy seeds, pumpkin seeds, sesame seeds, sunflower seeds | Include regularly in your eating habits, especially peanuts, chestnuts, walnuts and ground flaxseeds |

| Food Group | Foods to eat | Foods to avoid | Comments |
|---|---|---|---|
| Legumes and soya products | All beans except … | Aduki bean, black bean, black-eyed pea, fava bean, chick peas (garbanzos), kidney bean, lima bean, mung bean (sprouts) | Soya and haricot (navy) beans are the most beneficial beans for you |
| | Soya (bean, cheese, milk, miso, tempeh, tofu etc) | | Soya products are an excellent source of protein for you |
| Grains and related products | Amaranth, barley, couscous, Essene bread (100% sprouted grain bread), millet, oats, rice, rye, spelt, quinoa, wheat, wild rice | Buckwheat, corn, kamut, sorghum, tapioca | Avoid wheat if you have weight or respiratory problems |
| Vegetables | All except … | Artichoke (domestic, globe, Jerusalem), capers, chilli peppers, black olives, mushroom (abalone, shiitake), peppers (green, red, yellow), pickle (in brine, in vinegar), radish, radish sprouts, rhubarb | Make vegetables the "king" at your table |
| Fruits | All except … | Avocado, banana, bitter melon, coconut, dewberry, guava, mango, orange, persimmon, pomegranate, prickly pear, quince, starfruit | Eat about 450g/1lb of fruit per day. It has a cleansing effect |
| Spices | All except … | Anise, allspice, pepper (black, cayenne, white, peppercorns, red flakes) | Use turmeric and ginger on a regular basis for their digestive and anti-inflammatory effects |
| Culinary herbs | All | | Parsley is very good for ABs so eat it in large quantities and include flat-leaf parsley regularly in your salads |
| Beverages | Cider, green tea, lager, soda water, wine (red, white) | Coffee, spirits, fizzy drinks, tea (black) | Green tea should be your beverage of choice |

# soups

In China, soups represent the link between the art of eating and the art of healing. Often ingredients are carefully chosen to enhance the health of the recipient – it then becomes a real remedy. In everyday life, soups are also a precious health-giving brew. In fact traditional Chinese cooking in general is closely linked with health; something we are just beginning to put into practice in the West.

But back to the magical brew. It can contain whole pieces of meat, fish, poultry, herbs, vegetables, grains and beans, or the ingredients can be blended to achieve a smooth effect. And in addition to these main ingredients, don't forget that the use of stock instead of water also adds invaluable nutrients to your soup (see page 183 on how to make stocks).

You may use an endless combination of vegetables to make blended, stock-based soups. Each time you will end up with a different taste. This is a useful way of using up vegetables that are left in the bottom of the refrigerator. But don't just think of soups as a way of using up leftovers – they are a great way of using wonderfully fresh and colourful vegetables, so experiment. Try making a white soup with cauliflower, an orange soup with carrots, a dark green soup with leafy green vegetables and root tops, a red soup with tomatoes …

# Borsch

**Borsch is a traditional Russian soup made with a base of kale and beetroot (beet). Each region has its own recipe in which the additional ingredients vary. In this recipe, the vibrant red colour stands out even more once the cream and dill have been added.**

O replace the leeks with more onions and omit the cream

A omit the meat and replace the water with chicken stock for a more nutritious soup. Omit the pepper

B suitable

AB use lamb. Omit the pepper

SERVES 6–8

| | |
|---|---|
| 1½lb/675g raw beetroot (beet) | 1lb/450g leeks |
| 1 tbsp brown sugar | 8 cups/2 litres water |
| Juice of 1 lemon | 2lb/1kg lean stewing beef or lamb |
| 3 cups/750ml water | 1lb/450g kale |
| 2 tbsp olive oil | Sea salt and freshly ground black pepper |
| 1lb/450g onions | 1 cup/250ml sour cream |
| 5 garlic cloves | Fresh dill, finely chopped |
| ⅔lb/300g carrots | |

1. Slice the raw beetroot (beet) and cut into matchstick-size pieces.
2. Mix the sugar with the lemon juice and pour over the beetroot (beet). Leave to stand for 30 minutes. Transfer to a saucepan, cover with the 3 cups/750ml water, bring to the boil and cook for 30 minutes.
3. Heat the olive oil in a large saucepan, add the onions, garlic, carrots and leeks and sauté over medium heat until tender. Add the water and meat and cook for 1 hour.
4. Now shred the kale and add to the meat and vegetables along with the seasoning.
5. Drain the beetroot (beet) and set aside the juice. Add the beetroot (beet) to the borsch. Cook for 30 minutes.
6. Remove the meat, cut into bite-size pieces, and return it to the soup.
7. Just before serving, warm the beetroot (beet) juice but do not let it boil, and add it to the soup. Serve topped with sour cream and chopped dill.

## Ingredient Info: Kale

Kale is a variety of cabbage and as such is a member of the cruciferous family of vegetables. The others are broccoli, cauliflower, Brussels sprouts, turnips, collard greens and radishes. Cruciferous vegetables have been the object of scientific interest recently because their very high phytonutrient content means they have anti-cancer health benefits. Population studies have shown kale to be extensively consumed by those who have low rates of many types of cancer. However, the cruciferous family of foods also contain substances called goitrogens that can potentially interfere with the production of thyroid hormone. This seems only to be a problem if iodine is lacking in the diet. So, as ever, balance is the key.

Kale is a very rich source of carotenoids and chlorophyll. It is packed with vitamins and minerals and is considered to have the most beta carotene of all the green leafy vegetables. Surprisingly, one cup of kale can yield at least as much calcium as a cup of milk. This makes it useful for those of you who shouldn't be eating milk products or very little – Os and As.

Raw cabbage contains a substance – vitamin U – that helps soothe the gastrointestinal tract and heal stomach ulcers. Dr Garnett Cheney, professor at the University of Stanford, USA, successfully treated 95 out of 100 patients with gastric ulcers using raw cabbage juice. Since the publication of his work, cabbage juice has been recommended for gastrointestinal ulcers. If you are an O and are susceptible to or suffer from digestive ulcers, try consuming 2 cups/500ml fresh raw cabbage juice every day in divided doses for 6–8 weeks. The pain usually subsides within a few days.

The kale variety of cabbage may be eaten by all blood groups. Eat it raw, cooked and in juices. Make it a regular part of your diet.

# Broccoli Velouté

**This soup takes only 15 minutes to make. The courgette (zucchini) gives it a lovely smooth texture.**

O   suitable

A   omit the pepper

B   suitable

AB  omit the pepper

SERVES 4

1lb/450g broccoli

2 tbsp olive oil

2 medium onions, finely sliced

1 large courgette (zucchini), finely sliced

½ tsp sea salt

4 cups/1 litre boiling water or chicken stock

Freshly ground black pepper

2 tbsp chopped fresh parsley or chervil

Red peppercorns, optional

1.   Prepare the broccoli. Cut off the florets, peel off the hard skin on the stem and cut the stem into small pieces.
2.   Heat the oil in a large saucepan, add the onions and courgette (zucchini) and cook until the onions become translucent. Add the salt and the liquid. Add broccoli, cover, bring to the boil and cook for 10 minutes.
3.   Blend in a food processor or liquidizer.
4.   Season to taste and serve sprinkled with the chopped greenery and a few red peppercorns.

## Ingredient Info: Broccoli

As a member of the cruciferous family (see Borsch recipe), broccoli has potent anti-cancer properties. It also has the potential for inhibiting breast cancer. Indeed broccoli contains a compound – indole-3-carbinol – that helps the body excrete a form of estrogen associated with breast cancer (for which type As have a susceptibility). The same substance may also have a beneficial effect on prostate cancer.

# Chilled Avocado Soup

**You can either add ground ginger or curry powder to this recipe. Both choices are excellent and very different.**

O   not suitable

A   suitable

B   suitable

AB  not suitable

SERVES 4

3 medium avocado pears

3 cups/750ml apple juice

Juice of 1 lime

1 garlic clove, crushed

1 tsp ground ginger or curry powder, according to your choice

Sea salt to taste

½ lime cut in 4 fine slices, to garnish

1. Process all the ingredients in the food processor. Adjust the seasoning if necessary.
2. Refrigerate before serving.
3. Serve in individual soup bowls with a fine slice of lime in the middle.

## Ingredient Info: Avocado

Avocados are very rich in beneficial monounsaturated fat; similar to the type found in olive oil. They have been shown to reduce cholesterol by lowering LDL cholesterol – the "bad" type. They have also been shown to have antioxidant properties, due to a high glutathione content, thus further assuring cardiovascular protection.

Avocados contain appreciable amounts of vitamin E and more than double the amount of potassium than bananas.

In Asian countries avocado is recommended to soothe an inflamed digestive tract and duodenal ulcers. It also counteracts halitosis or bad breath resulting from unbalanced gut flora. However, avocado also contains a lectin that makes it unsuitable for Os and ABs.

# Chinese Chicken or Turkey Broth

**This Asian version of a chicken broth is lighter in texture and taste than the Western version. In China, chicken broth is appreciated for its health properties as it strengthens the body's energy – the *chi* or *qi*. As turkey is good for all blood groups, Bs and ABs can replace chicken with turkey.**

| O | suitable | B | use turkey |
|---|----------|---|------------|
| A | suitable | AB | use turkey |

SERVES 6

| | |
|---|---|
| 3½lb/1½kg chicken or turkey, cut into 10–12 pieces | 6 garlic cloves, unpeeled |
| 3 quarts/3 litres cold water | 9 green onions, trimmed |
| 6 slices of fresh ginger root | 1 tsp sea salt |
| | Fresh coriander (cilantro), to garnish |

1. Place the chicken or turkey pieces in a deep stainless steel stock pot. Bring to a slow boil, lower the heat and remove impurities that rise to the top. Continue the process as long as necessary. This will take approximately 30 minutes. Be sure not to let the stock boil during this time; it must only simmer. Simmering and skimming are the two essential steps for a clear stock.
2. Add the other ingredients, skim off any fat that appears on the surface, and leave to simmer for 2–4 hours.
3. Remove the ginger, garlic and green onions. Serve the broth with chicken or turkey pieces in individual bowls. Garnish with coriander (cilantro) leaves.

## Ingredient info: Stock

Read about the benefits of stock on page 183.

# Miso Soup

**This miso soup is our simplified and quick version of the Japanese classic.**

O    suitable

A    suitable

B    not suitable

AB   suitable

SERVES 1

---

1 cup/250ml boiling water or Vegetable Stock
(see page 186)

2 tsp miso

¼ garlic clove, crushed

¼ tsp grated fresh ginger root

1 tbsp finely chopped green onion

Coriander (cilantro) leaves, to garnish

1.  Heat the water or stock to boiling point.
2.  Place the miso in a bowl and add just enough water or stock to cream the miso. Add the rest of the liquid, then the garlic, ginger root and green onions.
3.  Garnish with coriander (cilantro) leaves. Serve immediately.

## Ingredient Info: Miso

Miso is a paste made from fermented soya beans or fermented soya beans with rice and barley. It can be used as the base for a Japanese-style soup or added to a vegetable soup to add flavour and depth. You may also add miso to flavour salad dressings, sauces, bean and vegetable dishes. When adding to a large amount of liquid such as a soup, put the miso in a small cup, add some of the broth from the soup, mix well to obtain a creamy texture, then add this to your soup. Miso should not be cooked as this will alter its flavour and beneficial health qualities.

For centuries the Japanese have considered miso to have an important role to play in longevity and good health. In more recent years, it has been the subject of scientific research in the East and West. The process of fermentation transforms the protein in miso in such a way that it is almost totally available to the body. It also inactivates the anti-nutrient factors in the raw soya beans. Miso, because of the lengthy fermentation, is a source of enzymes and beneficial lactic acid bacteria that are an aid to digestion. Miso's alkalizing effect is well known in Eastern Asia, where it is thought of as highly cleansing for the body.

In Japan they also found that a bowl of miso soup a day could lower the risk of stomach cancer. Among other reported effects are its antioxidant activity and the ability to lower cholesterol.

As and ABs should eat miso regularly to help prevent cardiovascular problems and cancer. Os can also benefit from miso but Bs should avoid it.

# legumes: beans and lentils

Legumes are an excellent source of protein for those of you whose blood group is A. Os and Bs are better off getting their main source of protein from meat, fish and poultry. ABs have their particular choice of beans, as do the other blood groups, and again can eat them as long as they don't rely on them alone for their source of protein.

Legumes have lots of good health benefits, so As in particular take note. Legumes have the ability to lower LDL cholesterol, the type that can clog up your arteries and cause heart disease. Beans, because of their high fibre content, contribute to lowering blood pressure. They also slow down the release of sugar in the blood and therefore the release of insulin. Dr J. Anderson, well known for his work on diabetes, has found that by eating beans, insulin-dependent diabetics were able to reduce their insulin by 38 per cent. If you are an A and have blood sugar problems, make sure you regularly include beans in your diet. This may prevent you from developing diabetes.

There is controversy regarding soya beans. Legumes contain substances called protease inhibitors that can block the action of our body's own digestive enzymes. Soya beans in particular can inhibit the protein digesting enzyme trypsin. Feeding animals raw soya meal has been shown to stunt their growth and increase the size of their pancreas, while stimulating the production of more enzymes. Some experts speculate that for humans, eating uncooked soya could generate enlargement of the pancreas and, in the long run, could reduce the production of enzymes. However, enzyme expert Dr Anthony J. Cichoke believes that cooking inactivates these protease inhibitors.

There is a positive aspect that probably largely outweighs these potential negative aspects, and that is the anti-cancer properties of protease inhibitors. Several researchers have found that when these substances were given to laboratory animals who should have developed cancer, they actually appeared to prevent the disease. Lignans, another substance in beans (and flaxseeds), are well known for their anti-cancer effects. The specific protease inhibitor in soya beans, according to Dr P. D'Adamo, may also protect against rheumatoid arthritis, endometriosis, inflammation and infections.

Beans contain phytates that also have a Jekyll and Hyde aspect to them. Phytates have been shown to bind minerals, making them less available to the body. But they also have been shown to have an anti-cancer effect. If you consume a diet rich in minerals derived from all sorts of sources, and don't rely solely on beans, then phytates shouldn't be a problem.

Our bodies require "complete" protein to function properly. Proteins are made of amino acids. There are over 20 different ones, of which eight are termed essential because our body cannot make them and needs to obtain them from the food we eat. The non-essential ones can be made from the essential amino acids.

Animal proteins are complete proteins because they contain all the essential amino acids. They also contain others. Legumes, with the exception of soya, lack two essential amino acids: lysine and methionine. By combining legumes with other foods that contain these essential amino acids you will not lack good healthy protein. Milk products, grains (spelt, rye, quinoa, millet, rice etc.) and nuts and seeds (walnuts, sesame seeds, pumpkin seeds, almonds etc.) complement legumes in this way. Some years ago it was thought that one needed to have these foods at the same meal. It now seems this is not necessary and as long as you combine them within a 48 hour period, your body will do the job of making the complete protein.

Legumes can be "noisy" once they hit the large intestine. This is because they contain oligosaccharides (several sugar molecules attached to each other) that are not digested by the enzymes in our small intestine. As soon as they reach the large intestine (colon) certain bacteria that have set up residence there will use these sugars as food, acting upon them and producing gas. This is what some people feel when they eat beans. It seems that if your intestinal flora is up to par you will be able to eat beans without being bothered in this way. If you are not used to eating beans, gradually increase your consumption and you should find your body will eventually accept them.

To reduce the gas-producing effect of beans ensure they are fresh – from the last harvest if possible. Also ensure that you soak the beans adequately (see page 188) as many of the oligosaccharides will be leached out with the soaking water. Soaking and lengthy cooking also eliminate most of the lectins present in beans.

# Black Turtle Bean Soup

**This soup is always greatly appreciated and looks so good with the green sauce in the middle.**

| | | | |
|---|---|---|---|
| O | suitable | B | not suitable |
| A | suitable | AB | not suitable |

SERVES 4

---

½lb/225g black turtle beans, soaked overnight (see page 188)

2 tbsp olive oil

1 tbsp cumin seeds

7 medium onions, finely sliced

2 pieces of fresh ginger root the size of a nutmeg

1 tsp dried thyme

1 tsp dried oregano

1 bay leaf

Fresh coriander (cilantro) stems from the sauce,

Fresh Coriander Sauce (see recipe on page 139)

1. Rinse the beans thoroughly.
2. Heat the olive oil in a heavy saucepan, add the cumin seeds and stir and cook until you smell a rich cumin aroma – about 30 seconds. Don't let the cumin burn as it will give off a bitter taste.
3. Add the onions and let them cook until they become translucent. Add the beans, ginger, thyme, oregano, bay leaf. Tie the coriander (cilantro) stems together with trussing string and add to the pan.
4. Cover the onions and beans with 2½ inches/7.5cm of water and bring to the boil. With a slotted spoon remove any froth that appears on the surface of the soup. Do not yet add the salt as it will toughen the beans. Cover the pan and simmer on a low heat for 2 hours. Add more water if necessary.
5. Remove two large ladles of beans and set aside. Remove the ginger, bay leaf and coriander (cilantro) stems and discard. Blend the soup. Return the unblended beans to the blended soup and sprinkle in the necessary salt.
6. Serve in individual soup plates with a tablespoon of the coriander (cilantro) sauce in the middle.

# Winter White Bean Soup

**This hearty soup is a meal in itself when served with just a slice of bread.**

O   use a hard sheep or goat's cheese

A   use a hard sheep or goat's cheese

B   use Parmesan (Parmigiano Reggiano)

AB  use a hard sheep or goat's cheese

SERVES 4

---

½lb/225g butter (lima) beans, soaked overnight (see page 188)

2 garlic cloves, sliced

1 fresh bouquet garni (with bay leaf, sage, rosemary and thyme)

3 tbsp olive oil

4 medium onions, thinly sliced

4 celery stalks, finely chopped

1 tsp sea salt

6 cups/1½ litres Vegetable or Chicken stock (see pages 186 and 184), or water

⅔lb/300g kabucha (golden hubbard, butternut or other winter squash) cut into ¾ inch/2cm squares

5 stalks swiss chard, leaves only, finely shredded

6 garlic cloves, freshly crushed just before serving

Extra virgin olive oil

Sea salt and freshly ground black pepper

Freshly grated cheese according to your blood group

1. Cover the beans in a large amount of water, add the garlic and the bouquet garni. Cook for 1¼ hours.
2. During this time prepare the vegetables. Heat the olive oil, add the onions, celery and salt. Sauté over low heat until vegetables become translucent, then cook for 5 minutes.
3. Remove the bouquet garni, heat the liquid and pour it over the vegetables. Add the squash, swiss chard leaves and beans. Cook for 10 minutes on a medium to low heat.
4. Just before serving, add the freshly crushed garlic.
5. At the table drizzle olive oil over the soup, add freshly ground black pepper and grated cheese according to your blood group.

# Fresh Bean and Onion Soup

Towards the end of summer and in the autumn cannellini (navy) beans can be found fresh, still in their pods. In this state they do not require soaking. You may also make this recipe with dried beans. You must, however, soak and cook them in the usual way (see page 188).

O   suitable

A   suitable

B   suitable

AB  suitable

SERVES 4

2lb/1kg fresh cannellini (navy) beans in their pods
2lb/1kg onions, cut into thin slices
2 tbsp olive oil
4 celery stalks
8 garlic cloves, cut in 2
2 sprigs of fresh savory
20 fresh sage leaves

4 cups/1 litre water
1 tbsp sea salt
Handful of celery leaves
Olive oil
Grated Parmigiano Reggiano or dry sheep's
    cheese

1.  Rinse the beans thoroughly.
2.  Sauté the onions in the oil until they become soft and slightly golden.
3.  Cut the celery stalks at a slant into ½ inch/1cm pieces and add them to the onions, along with the garlic. Sauté for a few minutes.
4.  Add the shelled beans, savory, sage and water. The liquid must just cover the vegetables and beans. Do not salt at this point as this will toughen the beans.
5.  Cook for 45 minutes to an hour until the beans are tender. Keep checking the liquid level, adding more if necessary. Fifteen minutes before the end, add the salt.
6.  Just before serving add the celery leaves, cut into thin strips. Divide the soup between individual soup bowls, drizzle with a little olive oil and sprinkle generously with grated cheese.

## Ingredient Info: Parmigiano Reggiano

Read about Parmigiano Reggiano cheese in the Pear, Walnut and Parmesan Salad on page 72, then decide whether you want to use it or the sheep cheese tolerated by all blood groups.

# salads

Many vegetables can be eaten raw as a salad and this is an excellent way of obtaining your vitamins and enzymes unaltered by cooking. According to oriental medicine it is best to eat more salads in the summer than in the winter, when one needs warming up from the inside.

Experiment with vegetables you would not normally think of eating raw: add some fresh green peas to a crunchy lettuce, grate raw courgette (zucchini) and young raw turnips, thinly slice raw cauliflower, make our raw fennel salad or spinach salad, grate celeriac and dress with a mayonnaise sauce. Even artichokes can be eaten raw. The Italians serve raw artichoke heart drizzled with lemon juice and olive oil. If you find that raw foods don't agree with you it may well be that your digestive system needs care. In this case, seek the help of a nutritionist.

The salads presented here are not exclusively made with raw ingredients, but the emphasis as always is on freshness. Make it a point to buy only the freshest ingredients and to use them promptly. And don't forget to use culinary herbs in abundance as they too provide valuable health benefits.

## culinary herbs

These herbs, well-known for adding a delicious taste and aroma to foods, also have health benefits. For thousands of years people have used herbs to treat their ailments, and for over 20 years now scientific research has been looking at their components in an attempt to understand how they work. Much is left to be done but we can no longer say there is no scientific proof for the virtues of herbs.

Culinary herbs are part of a long list of plants whose leaves, flowers, seeds, roots, bark and fruits can be used. By adding a generous amount of these aromatic plants to your diet your health will benefit. Almost every culinary herb acts on one or more aspects of digestion. This characteristic is of great interest to us here because it is not only what we eat that influences our health but first and foremost what we digest and absorb. You can buy organic produce and prepare your food with care, but if your digestive system is faulty, chronic disorders may result. Herbs in their many forms can be a great aid to digestion.

The herbs listed on the following pages should be used profusely – this will not only add zest to your salads, vegetables, meats, fish and fruit but will ensure the maximum digestive benefit. Experiment with the different herbs. Wash and dry them, snip off the leaves and, if necessary, tear or cut them into smaller bits.

## Parsley

Often parsley is used only to decorate our food. It is, however, very rich in carotenoids, flavonoids, folic acid, vitamin C, calcium and iron – all very precious nutrients. Its chlorophyll content is also very high. Parsley contains many other components and phytonutrients that, combined with its vitamins and minerals, give it valuable medicinal and curative properties.

In Roman times, parsley was used to increase the strength of the gladiators. It has a diuretic effect and is of assistance to the whole genito-urinary zone. It can help regulate menstrual cycles, bring on a delayed period and prevents the formation of gas in the stomach and intestines. It has a general pacifying effect on the digestive system. The high chlorophyll content of parsley neutralizes the smell of garlic in the mouth.

More recent studies have shown that parsley has protective effects against the carcinogenic potential of fried foods.

## Coriander (Cilantro) leaves

Coriander (cilantro) is native to the Mediterranean area and western Asia, but is now used in many cuisines. As a food, the leaves have a stimulating and tonic effect on digestion and help prevent flatulence. The medicinal use of the leaves and seeds is broader still: for dysentery, cholesterol, hepatitis and as a diuretic. The leaves and seeds stimulate the function of the kidneys and ease excessive menstrual flow. It is also known as an aphrodisiac. Coriander (cilantro) also helps neutralize garlic breath, so chew on some after a garlic-rich meal.

## Dill

Widely used nowadays in Scandinavian cooking, the medicinal value of dill leaves and seeds were known to ancient Egypt and Greece. In India today dill is used for many ailments. The seeds are an excellent remedy against flatulence and intestinal spasms, and chewing on them alleviates bad breath. The leaves stimulate digestion and at the same time have a calming effect. A teaspoonful of a decoction made from fresh dill leaves will relieve colic. In addition, its slight sedative effect can help promote sleep.

## Sweet Basil

Basil is a member of the mint family. It has a soothing effect on the digestive and the nervous systems. It relieves indigestion, promotes sleep and reduces nervousness, anxiety and irritability. It helps the function of the stomach by aiding in the release of gas, and relieving nausea and vomiting. It also helps in the expulsion of worms. Basil is a good disinfectant and can be a good remedy against migraine. Use basil extensively between April and October when it grows naturally and is at its sweetest.

## Mint

One of the most widely used aromatic herbs, mint is well known for its digestive properties: it relieves intestinal gas, gripping pains and nausea. Mint can stimulate the secretion of bile, which plays an essential role in the digestion of fat. With the help of digestive enzymes, bile emulsifies the fat we ingest – in other words it transforms large globules of fat into microparticles that are able to pass through the intestinal mucosa into the blood circulation to nourish our body. Bile is also necessary for the absorption of the fat soluble vitamins: A, D, E and K. Problems with bile can bring on constipation, intolerance to fats and bad breath. Several studies have shown that various components in mint could help dissolve gall bladder stones.

Mint has an antiviral effect and can therefore be used in case of fever, flu and the common cold. It also has a tonic effect on the nervous system, relieving anxiety and tension. Try an infusion of mint before going to bed to relax and calm yourself.

## Saffron

Saffron – the most expensive aromatic herb in the world – is made from the stigmas of the crocus flower. Each flower has three stigmas and approximately 150,000 are needed to make a pound of saffron. They can only be picked by hand, hence the high price. Luckily you only need a small amount to benefit from it. Saffron cultivated in Spain is the most prized. Avoid powdered saffron unless you are sure of its quality. In this form it soon loses its fragrance and taste and is easily adulterated.

As with most of the culinary herbs, saffron has beneficial effects on the digestive system. It eases the work of the stomach and combats flatulence and spasms. It has been used to bring on a delayed period, regulate the menstrual cycle and to ease period pains. It also has a reputation for increasing libido. The Romans and Greeks used it extensively as a remedy as well as a spice. Today, however, its cost means it is rarely used for its medicinal qualities. Other herbs can easily replace it.

## Sage

In the past sage was considered to be a sacred herb because of its enormous medicinal qualities. Its botanical name, salvia, comes from the latin word *salvare*, meaning to cure. Sage has a general stimulating effect on the body and is recommended for excessive fatigue and during convalescence. It is a natural tranquillizer and helps to balance the emotions.

Sage is also well known for its beneficial effects on mouth and throat infections, and as a gargle or mouthwash. It strengthens the gums and protects the teeth against gum recession. Sage has an anti-inflammatory effect and helps prevent mouth ulcers. Taken as an infusion, it helps combat infections – particularly of the urinary tract.

Sage is a great ally for women. It can help with heavy periods, increase fertility, reduce pain, and ease the symptoms of the menopause. In particular it helps reduce perspiration linked with hot flushes. Sage should be used carefully during pregnancy but taken towards the end, it can ease delivery.

## Tarragon

Termed the Queen of herbs, tarragon is native to Siberia, the Himalayas and North America. French tarragon, the variety used today, is a most outstanding herb with an energetic and highly aromatic licorice-like taste. It is particularly good for encouraging an appetite in those recovering from illness.

It can be used in cooked foods as well as in salads. Tarragon works wonders with chicken, rabbit and green salads. To make a highly aromatic vinegar let several tarragon stems steep in vinegar for six weeks. You can be more liberal with tarragon in cooking than in salads as it has a very penetrating taste when raw.

## Chervil

Delicate in touch and taste, chervil imparts its beautiful anise-like taste to the classic French *"omelette au cerfeuil"*, or omelette with chervil. The Greeks and Romans knew how to appreciate this herb. Unfortunately, its medicinal properties have been somewhat forgotten. Used in the spring it helps restore the body after a long winter of culinary abuses. Chervil is a tonic, diuretic and detoxifier and strengthens the body while cleansing it. Chervil also stimulates both the appetite and the digestion, and can be used as an eye wash to calm irritation.

## Bay leaf

As with many other herbs, bay leaf has a regulating effect on the stomach and upper intestine. It calms an irritated stomach and stimulates a lazy one by reviving the appetite and digestive juices. Used as an infusion after a meal, bay leaf contributes to good digestion and helps combat flatulence.

The dried leaves should be green; if yours are brownish replace them. Fresh leaves can also be used. They are stronger in taste and in order not to overwhelm your dish with bay leaves use half a leaf of fresh laurel where you would use a whole leaf of the dried herb. The bitterness of the fresh leaves disappears after a few days of drying.

Always remember to remove the leaf before serving a dish as its pointed shape and sharp edges could injure the throat.

# Beetroot Salad with Walnuts and Roquefort

**Use seasonal mixed green leaves for this salad. If you are preparing it in the spring, add young dandelion leaves.**

| O | suitable | B | suitable |
|---|----------|---|----------|
| A | omit the pepper | AB | omit pepper |

SERVES 4

8 small young red beetroot (beets), plus the small leaves for the salad

Mixed green salad i.e. oakleaf, rocket (arugula), escarole, chicory etc.

12 freshly shelled walnuts

5oz/150g roquefort cheese

3 tbsp cold pressed walnut oil

1 tbsp lemon juice

Sea salt and freshly ground black pepper

1. Steam the beetroot (beet) for 25–30 minutes. Using a sharp knife, test if they are done. Skin the beetroot (beets) and cut into thin slices.
2. Prepare the various salad leaves.
3. Break the walnuts up and cut the roquefort into large pieces.
4. Mix together the oil, lemon juice, salt and pepper.
5. Before serving, toss the salad leaves with the dressing and put them on individual salad plates. Add the beetroot (beet) slices, then the cheese and walnuts.

## Nutritional Info: Walnuts

The walnut is a very healthy nut. It is one of the few to contain linolenic acid – also called omega-3 oil. Our western diets lack this valuable family of oils and a variety of health problems are linked with this deficiency. Although walnuts are high in fat, they contain beneficial fats. They are also a good source of protein, minerals (calcium, magnesium, zinc, copper and selenium) and fibre.

In addition, walnuts have been shown to lower cholesterol by 18 per cent, when added to a low fat diet. People on the same diet minus the nuts only reduced their cholesterol by 6 per cent. You only need to eat one to two ounces of walnuts a day (30–60g or 5–10 nuts) to receive this benefit. Walnuts also have the ability to reduce toxicity in the body.

As walnuts are rich in linolenic acid they become rancid very easily and therefore should only be bought in their shells and cracked just before eating.

# Cucumber Raita with Grilled Cumin Seeds

Raita is an Indian dish of yogurt mixed with vegetables or fruit and various spices. It is a cooling dish and in Indian cuisine it is often served as an accompaniment to hot food. Cucumber raita can be served both as a salad and as a sauce – try it with the Gravlax (page 111) or Salmon Mousse (page 115).

| O | not suitable | B | suitable |
|---|---|---|---|
| A | suitable | AB | suitable |

SERVES 4

| | |
|---|---|
| I long cucumber, partially peeled and roughly grated | 2 cups yogurt (goat's, sheep's or cow's) |
| I tsp cumin seeds, roasted and ground | Sea salt |

1. Mix all the ingredients together and keep in the refrigerator until serving time.

## Ingredient Info: Cumin

Cumin seeds are commonly used in India, North Africa and Mexico, as well as in Middle Eastern cuisine. The medicinal properties of cumin mainly concern the digestive tract. Cumin relieves gas, bloating and spasms, acting as a relaxant to the gut. Simply place 1 teaspoon of cumin seeds in a cup of boiling water and let it infuse for 10 minutes.

Cumin seeds can also stimulate breast milk, and counteract insomnia and the common cold.

# Fennel Salad

**This simple and healthy salad will stimulate your digestive juices if eaten at the beginning of a meal.**

| | | | |
|---|---|---|---|
| O | suitable | B | suitable |
| A | suitable | AB | suitable |

SERVES 4

3 fennel bulbs

Juice of 1 lemon

½ bunch flat-leaf parsley, finely chopped

2 tbsp olive oil

Sea salt

1.  Discard the tough outer leaves of the fennel and keep the delicate greenery to garnish the salad.
2.  Cut the fennel into very fine slices – a mandoline can be useful here.
3.  As you cut the bulbs, pour a little lemon juice over them to stop oxidation. Place the fennel slices in a bowl and add the parsley, olive oil and salt.
4.  Check the seasoning and adjust if necessary. Decorate with the fennel greenery and serve.

## Ingredient Info: Fennel

Fennel is a typical Mediterranean vegetable and the Italians in particular make big use of it. The bulb is known to be helpful in digestive complaints such as slow digestion, intestinal spasms and flatulence.

# Fish, Rice, Baby Spinach Leaf and Red Onion Salad

**The secret of this recipe is in the individual preparation of the fish, rice and greenery. Each element can be prepared in advance and then brought together at the last moment.**

O   use vinegar-free mustard

A   use vinegar-free mustard

B   suitable

AB   use vinegar-free mustard

SERVES 4

---

1¾lb/780g white-fleshed fish such as cod or monkfish

½ cup/120g basmati rice

Fish stock (see page 185)

Juice of ½ a lime

1 bouquet dill, leaves chopped

3 tbsp extra virgin olive oil

2 tbsp lemon juice

2 tsp Dijon mustard

Sea salt and freshly ground black pepper

½lb/225g baby spinach leaves

1 large red onion, cut into very fine circles

½ bouquet fresh coriander (cilantro), stems discarded

1. Cook the rice in a large quantity of salted water for 15 minutes. Check that the grains remain firm. Rinse and leave to cool in a colander.

2. At the same time, either steam the fish above the fish stock, or poach it in the fish stock. The liquid must simmer and never boil. Let the fish cook for 15–30 minutes, according to the size of the fish. Let it cool in the liquid. Remove skin and bones and break into large pieces. Pour the lime juice over the fish and sprinkle it with fresh dill.

3. Mix the olive oil, lemon juice, mustard, salt and pepper. Drizzle half of the dressing over the rice and keep the other half for the spinach leaves.

4. When you are ready to serve, toss the spinach with the remaining dressing in a serving bowl, place the rice in the middle, add the fish on the sides, scatter the red onion slices over the fish and spinach and sprinkle the coriander (cilantro) leaves on top. Serve immediately. You may also arrange the salad directly on individual plates.

# Green Bean Salad with Basil

O  suitable

A  omit the tomatoes

B  omit the tomatoes

AB suitable

SERVES 4

Fresh basil leaves, to your taste

2 garlic cloves, crushed

Sea salt

3–4 tbsp extra virgin olive oil

1½lb/675g small thin green beans

2 medium tomatoes, peeled, seeded and diced or cherry tomatoes

1. Start by preparing the dressing. Wash the basil leaves and dry them with a paper towel. Tear the leaves into large pieces.
2. Put the basil, garlic and salt in a bowl and add the olive oil. Set aside to marinate.
3. Rinse the green beans, cut off the ends and pull off any strings.
4. Blanch the green beans in a large quantity of water for approximately 10 minutes; they should be *al dente* and very green. Stop the cooking by pouring the beans into a colander and rinsing them in cold water. This retains their beautiful green colour.
5. Once the beans are well drained but still warm, add the marinated olive oil dressing and toss well.
6. Serve the salad on individual plates topped with the tomatoes. Garnish with extra basil leaves.

## Ingredient Info: Basil

Basil comes in many different varieties so colour, taste and leaf size can vary. The amount used in a recipe depends on your sensitivity to the aroma. Read more about basil on page 63.

# Lentil Salad with Fennel and Herbs

| O | not suitable | B | not suitable |
|---|---|---|---|
| A | suitable | AB | suitable |

SERVES 4

¾lb/350g green lentils, rinsed and picked over
Juice of 1 lemon
6 tbsp extra virgin olive oil
1 tsp vinegar-free mustard
Sea salt

1 fennel bulb, finely sliced
1 bunch green onions, chopped
1 bunch parsley, chopped
1 bunch coriander (cilantro), chopped

1. Pour cold water over the lentils and bring to the boil. Drain, cover with water again and bring to the boil. Reduce the heat and simmer for 20 minutes until tender but slightly firm. They must hold their shape. Drain well.
2. Mix the lemon juice, olive oil, mustard and salt in a salad bowl. Incorporate the lentils and let them marinate in the dressing.
3. Just before serving add the fennel, onions, parsley and coriander (cilantro). Toss well.

## Ingredient Info: Lentils

See the information on Legumes: Beans and Lentils on pages 56–57.

# Marinated Grilled Peppers

**This Mediterranean classic is a favourite summer dish.**

O   suitable

A   not suitable

B   suitable

AB  not suitable

SERVES 4

---

6 (bell) peppers; 3 red, 3 yellow

3 tbsp fresh lemon juice

6 tbsp extra virgin olive oil

1 garlic clove, crushed

Sea salt and freshly ground black pepper

Fresh basil to taste

1. Cut the (bell) peppers in two and remove the core and seeds. Place the halves skin-side up on a baking sheet and grill (broil). Allow the skins to char, then remove from the baking sheet and leave to cool. Remove the skins.
2. Make the dressing by mixing the lemon juice, 4 tablespoons of olive oil, garlic and salt.
3. Cut each (bell) pepper half into 4 strips, lay them out on an earthenware dish and pour over the olive oil dressing.
4. Let the (bell) peppers marinate for several hours. Before serving, drizzle with the remaining olive oil, grind over some black pepper and garnish with fresh basil leaves.

## Nutritional Info: (Bell) Peppers

Peppers are an excellent source of nutrients and the red ones, in particular, are nutrient dense. They are especially high in vitamin C.

Peppers belong to the nightshade family and can aggravate arthritis in susceptible individuals. If you are a sufferer, try avoiding them to see if your condition improves.

# Pear, Walnut and Parmesan Salad

O   suitable

A   suitable

B   suitable

AB  suitable

SERVES 4

---

1 red or green oakleaf lettuce

Zest and juice of 1 non-treated lemon

2 ripe pears

20 walnuts

3 tbsp walnut oil

Sea salt

Fresh shavings of Parmigiano Reggiano or hard Italian sheep's cheese

Flat-leaf parsley or coriander (cilantro)

1. Remove the central stem from each lettuce leaf and tear the leaves into bite-size pieces.
2. Mix the lemon zest with the lemon juice.
3. Peel the pears, cut them in 4 and then cut lengthwise into slices. As you cut the fruit, pour a little lemon juice over the slices to stop the oxidation.
4. Shell the walnuts, aiming for perfect halves.
5. Mix the oil, the rest of the lime juice and the salt.
6. Just before serving toss the salad in the dressing, then divide it between individual serving plates. Decorate each salad with the pears, walnuts and the fresh cheese shavings.
7. Finish off with either the leaves of parsley or coriander (cilantro) or both. Serve immediately.

## Ingredient Info: Parmigiano Reggiano

This very special cheese is the authentic Parmesan cheese – made in Northern Italy in a very precise area around Parma and Reggio Emilia. According to specialists in Italy it has unusual health qualities for a cheese. Nutritionists in Italy recommend it for babies, children, the elderly and those concerned about their weight, as it is easily digestible and does not lie heavily on the stomach.

The fermentation method of Parmigiano Reggiano metabolizes the lactose and galactose in the curd meaning there is none left in the cheese. This may contribute to its reputed digestibility.

And what about the blood groups? The blood group researchers have apparently only tested "parmesan". Parmigiano Reggiano is different, it is not the same product. Hopefully one day we shall have the answer. In the meantime just give it a taste and see for yourself – it's outstanding.

# Quinoa Tabbouleh

Tabbouleh is a Lebanese dish made with bulgur, a sprouted precooked hard wheat. We wanted to make this dish without the wheat, which so many people should avoid, so we chose quinoa instead. Tabbouleh is full of vitamins due to the large quantity of parsley.

| | | | |
|---|---|---|---|
| O | suitable | B | omit the tomatoes |
| A | omit the tomatoes and pepper | AB | omit the pepper |

SERVES 4

---

¼lb/115g quinoa

Juice of 1 lemon

Extra virgin olive oil, same volume as the lemon juice

Sea salt and freshly ground black pepper

2 large bunches flat-leaf parsley, roughly chopped

4 tbsp fresh mint, finely chopped

½ bunch green onions, with their greenery finely chopped

2 tomatoes, peeled, seeded and diced

1. Rinse the quinoa. Boil double the amount of water to the volume of rinsed quinoa. Throw in the quinoa, add salt and cook for 10 minutes. The grain is cooked when you see a small white inner particle, the germ. Set aside to cool.
2. While the quinoa is cooking, mix the lemon juice, olive oil, salt and pepper to make the dressing.
3. Now chop the parsley, mint, onions and tomatoes. Mix them in the salad bowl, add the dressing, then the cooled quinoa. Allow time for the dressing to be absorbed by all the ingredients then adjust the seasoning if necessary. Serve.

## Nutritional Info: Quinoa

Quinoa was considered a sacred food by the Incas, who called it the "mother grain". After the arrival of the Spanish conquistadors quinoa was banished because of the supernatural powers attributed to it. Thanks to its unusual hardiness and ability to grow in desert-like areas, quinoa is enjoying a new life in South America and in many other countries.

Quinoa contains at least 16 per cent protein with a good quantity of lysine, methionine and cystine – amino acids lacking in other grains. It is therefore considered a complete protein. Quinoa is rich in highly digestible fatty acids and the minerals phosphorus, calcium and iron.

# Raw Beetroot Salad

**This is a simple, delicious and colourful salad – a delight for the eye and palate.**

| | | | |
|---|---|---|---|
| O | suitable | B | suitable |
| A | omit the pepper | AB | omit the pepper |

SERVES 4

---

| | |
|---|---|
| 2 large red beetroot (beets) | 1 garlic clove, crushed |
| 1 tbsp walnut oil | 1 tsp vinegar-free mustard |
| 20 walnuts in their shells | Sea salt and freshly ground black pepper |
| 3 tbsp olive oil | ¼lb/115g mixed green salad |
| 1 tsp lemon juice | |

1. Grate the beetroot (beets) with a very fine grater. Add the walnut oil.
2. Shell the walnuts yourself; they are so much better when fresh.
3. Mix the olive oil, lemon juice, garlic, mustard, salt and pepper for the dressing.
4. Just before serving, toss the green salad with the dressing, and place on 4 individual plates. In the middle of each plate arrange some of the raw beetroot (beet) mixture. Sprinkle the freshly broken walnuts over the salad.

## Nutritional Info: Beetroot (beet)

Beetroot (beet) is a very valuable food. It should be eaten regularly either cooked, raw or juiced. If you can get beetroot (beet) with their green leaves don't discard them. They contain even more valuable nutrients than the root. Use them in juices or salads, or cook them as you would spinach or in combination with spinach.

Beetroot (beet) has been used as a blood builder by naturopathic healers. Although it does not contain a very high amount of iron, it is present in a very absorbable form. Beetroot (beet) increases peristalsis, the wavelike movements of the bowel, thereby preventing constipation.

# Spinach Salad in Walnut Oil

**For this recipe we used an oil which has been extracted from grilled walnuts. Made by traditional methods in the walnut-growing regions in France, it is a joy to the palate.**

| | | | |
|---|---|---|---|
| O | use lemon juice | B | suitable |
| A | use lemon juice and omit the pepper | AB | use lemon juice and omit the pepper |

SERVES 4

| | |
|---|---|
| I tsp vinegar-free Dijon mustard | Sea salt and freshly ground black pepper |
| 3 tbsp walnut oil | I hard-boiled organic egg |
| I tbsp balsamic vinegar or lemon juice | ½lb/225g baby spinach leaves |

1. Make the salad dressing at the bottom of a salad bowl. First put in the mustard, then, stirring constantly, slowly add the oil, vinegar or lemon juice, salt and pepper.
2. Mash the hard-boiled egg with a fork.
3. Wash and dry the spinach leaves. Place the leaves in the salad bowl. Sprinkle the chopped egg over the salad.
4. Toss the salad just before serving.

## Ingredient Info: Spinach

Raw spinach has the ability to stimulate peristalsis of the bowel, meaning it encourages the wave-like movements of the intestine. It is a good remedy for constipation and sluggish elimination. This is due to the presence of organic oxalic acid. However, as soon as spinach is cooked the oxalic acid becomes inorganic and loses its ability to have this effect. Eat spinach as a salad as often as you can in the spring and summer when you can find young tender leaves, and add spinach to fresh vegetable juices.

Read more about spinach in the recipe for Spinach with Currants and Pine Nuts on page 94.

# Tofu Salad

**Many people seem to get discouraged with tofu. If this applies to you, try this recipe – it's one of the simplest ways of preparing it. No cooking is involved and you can vary the flavours by adding different herbs and spices to the marinade. This makes an excellent appetizer or light dinner.**

O   suitable

A   omit the pepper

B   not suitable

AB  omit the pepper

SERVES 4

½lb/225g tofu cut in ½ inch/1cm cubes
4 carrots
Salad leaves – oakleaf, romaine etc.
1 bunch coriander (cilantro)

MARINADE:
4 tbsp tamari or soya sauce
1 inch/2.5cm cube of fresh ginger root, finely
   grated

1 garlic clove, diced
1 pinch curry or turmeric powder

SALAD DRESSING:
3 tbsp extra virgin olive oil
1 tbsp lemon juice
Sea salt and freshly ground black pepper

1. Mix the marinade ingredients together and marinate the tofu cubes in the sauce for at least 30 minutes, preferably more, stirring from time to time so that it penetrates the bean curd.
2. Grate the carrots very finely – there is a world of difference between fine and rough grating.
3. Prepare the salad leaves of your choice.
4. When ready to serve, mix the dressing and toss with the salad in a large salad bowl. Distribute the salad on the individual plates, then lightly scatter over the grated carrots. Now sprinkle over the coriander (cilantro), then the tofu. Pour any remaining sauce over the salad.

# Curried Tomato Salad

**This can be served both as a salad and a sauce with the Salmon Mousse on page 115.**

O   suitable

A   not suitable

B   not suitable

AB  omit the pepper

SERVES 4

---

1lb/450g ripe tomatoes

1 cup/225g unsweetened soya yogurt

1 tbsp olive oil

2 tbsp finely chopped fresh flat-leaf parsley

1 shallot, finely chopped

1 tsp curry powder

Sea salt and freshly ground black pepper

1. Place the tomatoes into boiling water for 1 minute, then remove and set aside to cool. Peel the tomatoes, remove the seeds and dice the pulp.
2. In a bowl mix the soya yogurt, olive oil, parsley, shallot and curry powder. Add the tomatoes and season with salt and pepper. Serve immediately or refrigerate until serving time.

# Winter Salad with Walnuts, Prunes and Dried Apricots

**For this salad use mixed winter green leaves. The more variety it includes, the more colourful and appetizing it will be.**

O  suitable

A  omit the pepper

B  suitable

AB  omit the pepper

SERVES 4

Flat-leaf parsley, stems removed

Winter salad leaves (endive, radicchio, lamb's lettuce, etc.)

3 tbsp walnut oil

1 tbsp lemon juice

Sea salt and freshly ground black pepper

8 dried prunes

8 dried apricots

12 freshly shelled walnuts

1.  Prepare the parsley and salad leaves.
2.  Mix together the oil, lemon juice, salt and pepper for the dressing.
3.  Cut the prunes and apricots lengthwise into medium-sized slices.
4.  Break the walnuts into large pieces.
5.  Just before serving, toss the salad leaves with the dressing and put on individual salad plates. Add the prune and apricot slices and finish off with the walnuts.

# vegetables

We should all eat plenty of vegetables, irrespective of our blood type. Scientific research has recently been investigating various foods, and vegetables in particular, in order to understand their impact on different aspects of our health. Researchers are finding that certain substances in vegetables have a strong influence on the way our cells function, and thus affect the very basis of our health.

What scientists are discovering is that in addition to the nutrients that the body requires to stay alive (protein, carbohydrates, lipids, vitamins, minerals, amino acids and essential fatty acids), vegetables also contain substances that have health-enhancing effects as far reaching as protecting and fighting against cancer. These substances are called phytochemicals. Hundreds have been discovered and perhaps thousands more are out there waiting for scientific scrutiny. Major institutions, such as the National Cancer Institute in the US, now recommend eating at least three to five servings of vegetables every day. Top of the list for the cancer-fighting substances it contains is broccoli.

Another major benefit of both fresh and carefully cooked vegetables (and fruit) is the large amounts of antioxidants they contain. An important theory links ageing and disease with the process of oxidation taking place in the body. Oxygen is a vital nutrient that gives life to our cells, but it can also promote destruction. Oxidation in our bodies can be compared to the rusting of iron when it comes in contact with air (oxygen). Oxygen activity that is not controlled by "antioxidants" has a destructive effect on the cells of our body and consequently on the tissues and organs. Some researchers now believe that the major cause of illness and disease is the lack of protection against this oxidative damage.

This potential damage can be countered when the body is well equipped with natural inborn antioxidant mechanisms and antioxidant nutrients. These antioxidant nutrients are mainly found in fruit and vegetables. Beta carotene; vitamins A, C and E; and the minerals zinc, selenium, copper and manganese are the best known, but there are many others.

So eat your vegetables – they are one of the best forms of health insurance you can buy. Choose them fresh and in season, and avoid those that have come half way around the world. Eat them raw and cooked but avoid leftovers. Prepare just enough for the meal you are going to eat. Leftovers are not worth much and lack that special something that a freshly-prepared meal has. The Caucasian inhabitants, known for their centenarians, place great value on the freshness of their food. They chop their vegetables, grind their spices and cut their herbs just before using them – and they throw away their leftovers!

# Braised Carrots

**Serve these provençal-style carrots as they are or purée them and sprinkle with parsley.**

O   suitable

A   omit the pepper

B   suitable

AB   omit the pepper

SERVES 4

---

2lb/1kg carrots, cut in short sticks 2½ inches/6cm long

2 tbsp olive oil

1 tsp dried thyme

1 garlic bulb, separated and cloves peeled

Sea salt and freshly ground black pepper

Fresh flat-leaf parsley, finely chopped

1. Place the carrots and olive oil in a heavy saucepan and sauté until the carrots are coated in oil.
2. Add the thyme and peeled garlic cloves.
3. Add enough water to cover the carrots by ¼ inch/5mm and let them cook gently for 30 minutes. Check the water very regularly, adding more if necessary as carrots burn easily.
4. Drain the carrots if necessary, season and serve sprinkled with the parsley.

## Ingredient Info: Carrots

If your carrots are organic, don't peel them; most of the vitamins and the taste are just under the skin. If they have been treated, peel them to remove the pesticide residue.

Eating carotene-rich foods can protect against a variety of cancers. If you are or were a smoker, make it a point to eat an orange-coloured vegetable every day such as carrots, pumpkin, squash or sweet potatoes. Dark green leaves are also rich in carotenoids. Their green colour comes from the chlorophyll that masks the orange and yellow in them. See following page for more information on carrots.

# Braised Carrots, Fennel and Onions

| | | | |
|---|---|---|---|
| O | suitable | B | suitable |
| A | omit the pepper | AB | omit the pepper |

SERVES 4

---

| | |
|---|---|
| 1 lb/450g carrots | 1 medium onion, cut into very fine slices |
| 2 fennel bulbs | Sea salt and freshly ground black pepper |
| Olive oil | 1 bunch flat-leaf parsley, finely chopped |

1. Cut the carrots into very fine slices, preferably using a mandoline.
2. Cut the fennel in two lengthwise and continue cutting finely in the same direction so that the individual pieces remain attached to the central core.
3. Drizzle a little olive oil on the bottom of a heavy cast iron casserole, add the onions and half of the carrots, more olive oil, salt, the remaining carrots and finally the fennel. Drizzle over more olive oil if needed, and add salt and pepper.
4. Place greaseproof (waxed) paper, cut to the size of the casserole, on top of the vegetables and then cover. Cook slowly over low heat for 25–30 minutes. Test the carrots with a sharp knife
5. Serve sprinkled with parsley. The onions will slightly caramelize and the carrots will melt in the mouth.

## Ingredient Info: Carrots

Carotenoids – a family of nutrients found in dark green, yellow and orange vegetables such as kale, carrots, spinach, sweet potatoes, squash, tomatoes, corn, apricots, green and red (bell) peppers, and chard – have been shown by extensive research to offer some protection against cancer. The well-known beta carotene is one of them. Research at the Institute of Food Research in Norwich (UK) has recently shown that by cooking carrots or mashing them the carotenoids are made much more available for use by the body than if you eat them raw. Also, beta carotene is not destroyed by cooking. So eat cooked carrots as well as raw ones. When it comes to eating your carrots raw, why not try juicing them – this provides plenty of those valuable enzymes and breaking them down means you get more of the carotenoids. This also applies to the other vegetables listed above. Eat plenty of this valuable group of vegetables.

# Braised Fennel Bulbs

**This very Italian vegetable is an excellent accompaniment to fish, as well as lamb.**

O   suitable

A   omit the pepper

B   suitable

AB   omit the pepper

SERVES 4

2 tbsp olive oil

8 small fennel bulbs, trimmed, or 4 large ones cut
    into quarters

I tbsp thyme

Sea salt and freshly ground black pepper

Fennel leaves for garnishing

1. In a large cast iron casserole heat the olive oil, add the fennel and braise on all sides.
2. Add enough water just to cover the bottom of the casserole, then sprinkle with thyme, salt and pepper, cover, and cook on a low heat. Make sure there is always a little liquid at the bottom of the pan. Let the fennel cook for at least one hour until tender. Test with a knife.
3. Top with some of the finely chopped green leaves.

## Ingredient Info: Fennel

Fennel is a typical Mediterranean vegetable, and one that Italians make big use of. The bulb is known to ease digestive complaints such as slow digestion, intestinal spasms and flatulence. Eating fennel raw at the beginning of a meal is a good way to perk up your appetite. (See recipe for Fennel Salad page 67.)

# Broccoli with Garlic and Ginger

Often broccoli is overcooked, with the result that it loses its vibrant green colour and acquires a rather strong taste. This method of cooking broccoli keeps most of the nutrients intact.

| O | suitable | B | suitable |
| A | suitable | AB | suitable |

SERVES 4

| 1lb/450g broccoli | ¼ cup/60ml water |
| 1 tbsp olive oil | Sea salt |
| 8 garlic cloves, cut into slices | 1 tbsp grilled (broiled) sesame seeds, optional |
| 2 pieces fresh ginger root, size of nutmeg, cut into julienne strips | |

1. Cut the large stem off the broccoli. Peel the skin by pulling it away, then cut the stem into ½ inch/1cm pieces. Cut the florets in bite-size pieces.
2. Heat the oil in a large sauté pan. Add garlic, ginger and broccoli. Stir fry for a few seconds without letting the ingredients brown. Add water and salt. Cover.
3. Let the broccoli cook for 5–8 minutes, depending on the size of the florets and the quality of the broccoli. Check with a knife and add more water if necessary. The broccoli should retain a bit of crunch.
4. Serve immediately otherwise the broccoli will continue cooking.

## Ingredient Info: Broccoli

Read about broccoli in the recipe for Broccoli Velouté on page 52.

# Celeriac Purée with Parsley

**This very healthy purée is the perfect accompaniment to game and Christmas turkey. It has a beautiful green colour that complements the bright red of cranberry sauce.**

O    suitable

A    omit the pepper

B    suitable

AB    omit the pepper

SERVES 4

2lb/1kg celeriac root, cut into 1 inch/2.5cm cubes

1 large bunch flat-leaf parsley without stems

2 tbsp olive oil or clarified butter
    (see recipe page 187)

Sea salt

Freshly ground black pepper

1. Steam the celeriac for 20 minutes. Test with a sharp knife.
2. Add the parsley and steam for another 5 minutes.
3. Blend the celeriac and parsley in food processor, adding olive oil or clarified butter, salt and pepper. Serve immediately.

## Ingredient Info: Parsley

Read about parsley in the section on culinary herbs on page 62.

# Aubergine with Garlic and Thyme

O  suitable
A  not suitable

B  suitable
AB  omit the pepper

SERVES 4

---

1½lb/675g aubergine (eggplant)
3 tbsp extra virgin olive oil
12 garlic cloves, cut into slices
3 tbsp water

3 pinches thyme, preferably fresh
Sea salt and freshly ground black pepper
Flat-leaf parsley, freshly chopped

1. Cut the aubergines (eggplants) lengthwise into four, then cut into ½ inch/1cm slices horizontally.
2. Slowly heat the olive oil in a casserole, add the garlic and stir to prevent the pieces browning. Add the aubergine (eggplant).
3. Once all the oil is absorbed add the water, thyme and salt.
4. Continue cooking, adding more water if necessary so that the aubergine (eggplant) does not stick to the bottom of the casserole but remains moist. Allow 15 minutes cooking time.
5. Before serving sprinkle with parsley and freshly ground black pepper.

## Ingredient Info: Aubergine (eggplant)

The aubergine (eggplant) is native to India, where it grows in many different shapes, sizes and colours. It has been considered a "health food" in Asia for thousands of years. Research has shown that aubergine (eggplant) prevents blood cholesterol levels from rising after eating a meal containing fat. It also has digestive properties due to its stimulating effect on the pancreas and the liver.

Aubergine (eggplant) is a member of the nightshade family and as such can aggravate arthritis in sensitive people.

# End-of-Holiday Vegetables

We put this vegetable dish together at the end of a cooking session to use up our leftover vegetables. Use whichever ones you might have left over to make a similar dish.

| O | suitable | B | suitable |
|---|---|---|---|
| A | omit the pepper | AB | omit the pepper |

---

Celery, cut at a slant into 2 inch/5cm pieces

Courgette (zucchini), cut lengthwise in four, then at a slant into 2 inch/5cm pieces

Leeks, cut in two then at a slant into 2 inch/5cm pieces

2 slices fresh ginger root, cut into matchsticks

Olive oil

Sea salt and freshly ground black pepper

1. Cook all the vegetables in a wok with the ginger and olive oil. The key to this recipe is in the cutting.

## Ingredient Info: Celery

Read about celery in Super Vegetable Juice for Group A page 166.

# Green Peas and Green Onions

Fresh green peas from the pod are delicious. Eat them as soon as possible after they have been picked, otherwise you are better off eating frozen peas. Soon after they are picked the natural sugars start converting to starch and the taste is just not the same – they become mealy. Freezing peas soon after picking halts this process. Every minute you put into shelling peas is worth it for the gastronomic payback.

| | | | |
|---|---|---|---|
| O | suitable | B | suitable |
| A | avoid the butter | AB | avoid the butter |

SERVES 4

1lb/450g green onions
2lb/1kg green peas in their pods
2 fresh rosemary sprigs
2 bay leaves

Water or Chicken Stock (see recipe page 184)
Sea salt and freshly ground black pepper
Olive oil, butter or clarified butter
   (see recipe page 187)

1. Prepare the onions by removing the roots and trimming off the greenery. Shell the peas.
2. Place the onions, rosemary, bay leaves, salt and pepper in 1 inch/2.5cm of water or chicken stock and simmer for 5 minutes.
3. Add the peas, cover and cook for 10 minutes. Be sure there is always a little liquid at the bottom of the pan. Test the softness of the onions; if tender turn off the heat. If the onions are cooked, the peas are cooked.
4. Drain if necessary, season and serve warm with a little olive oil, butter or clarified butter.

## Ingredient Info: Peas

Peas were first eaten as a dried food. The French discovered how tasty fresh peas were – they passed them around raw as a delicacy at the court of Louis XIV in the 17th century. Peas in France are known to act like a broom in the intestines. They are very easy to digest.

# Onion Pancakes

**Onions are a very healthy food and should be used as a vegetable in their own right. These pancakes make an excellent vegetable accompaniment to a meat dish or can be served as a light meal with a green salad and some goat's cheese.**

O   suitable                          B   suitable

A   omit the pepper                   AB  omit pepper

SERVES 4

---

1lb/450g onions, finely sliced        Sea salt and freshly ground black pepper

2 organic eggs                        Clarified butter (see recipe page 187)

2 tbsp spelt flour                    or olive oil

1.  Mix the onions, eggs, flour, salt and pepper in a bowl.
2.  Heat a little clarified butter in a frying pan (skillet) and add 1 tablespoon of the onion mixture. With the back of a fork flatten the pancake. Make as many pancakes as the frying pan (skillet) can hold. Let the pancakes cook and become golden before flipping them over. Again wait for the pancakes to become golden. Keep in a warm oven until serving time.

## Ingredient Info: Onions

Research in India has shown that as little as a tablespoon of onion a day can bring down your blood cholesterol. In addition, onions can help reduce the blood's tendency to clot. In other words onions are a great friend of your cardiovascular system. The more you eat, the greater the effect. Eat them both raw and cooked. Types A and AB should eat onions every day.

Onions are a rich source of quercetin, a flavonoid recommended in allergic and inflammatory conditions. Type Os, who have a tendency towards inflammatory diseases (arthritis) and allergies (asthma and hay fever), should eat plenty of red and yellow onions as these have the most quercetin. The good news is that it is not destroyed by cooking.

# Oven Fries

Who doesn't love delicious French fries every now and then? This version uses a very small amount of fat compared to the classic method of making them. To add extra flavour try adding dried thyme, oregano, savory or paprika. Add the herbs or spice before tossing the potatoes in the olive oil or clarified butter.

O   not suitable                          B   suitable
A   not suitable                          AB  omit the pepper

SERVES 4

---

4 large baking potatoes                   Sea salt and freshly ground pepper
2 tbsp olive oil or melted clarified butter
   (see recipe page 187)

1. Preheat the oven to 200°C/400°F/Gas mark 6.
2. Peel the potatoes – unless they are organic – and rinse. The rinsing is important as it helps remove the starch and prevents the potatoes sticking. Dry them.
3. Cut the potatoes lengthwise into long thin matchsticks ¼ inch/5mm thick. Toss the potatoes in the olive oil or clarified butter.
4. Place the fries on a large sheet of greaseproof (waxed) paper on a baking sheet and put them in the oven. Bake for 15–20 minutes until they become golden on the bottom, turn them over and bake for another 10–15 minutes until they become golden all over. Sprinkle with salt and serve.

# Roasted Winter Vegetables

O   suitable

A   omit the pepper

B   suitable

AB  omit the pepper

SERVES 6

---

12 small white and purple turnips – about 300g

1lb/450g carrots

10 small onions – about 300g

2 tbsp olive oil

Sea salt and freshly ground black pepper

2 sprigs of fresh rosemary, preferably fresh

1 garlic bulb, cloves peeled

1. Preheat the oven to 200°C/400°F/Gas mark 6.
2. Peel all the vegetables. Cut the turnips in two lengthwise and cut each half in three pieces.
3. Cut the carrots in two lengthwise if they are large, and then cut at a slant into 2 inch/5cm pieces
4. In a large bowl place the carrots, onions, and turnips, and pour over the olive oil. Mix well with your hands. Now add salt and pepper. Add the rosemary leaves.
5. In a large roasting pan spread out the vegetables so they are not on top of each other.
6. Roast for 30 minutes. After 15 minutes add the garlic cloves. Don't stir. The carrots, turnips and onions will slightly caramelize in the pan – this gives the vegetables their special taste.

# Saffron Potatoes in Lemon Juice

**These beautiful yellow potatoes are a delight to all who taste them.**

| | | | |
|---|---|---|---|
| O | not suitable | B | suitable |
| A | not suitable | AB | suitable |

SERVES 4

---

1 tsp/0.2 g saffron strands crushed with a spoon in 1 tablespoon of warm water

Juice of 2 lemons

3 tbsp olive oil

1¼lb/560g Roseval or similar potatoes that will not fall apart when cooked

Sea salt

1. Mix the saffron strands with the lemon juice and olive oil, and pour into an ovenware dish.
2. Peel the potatoes, cut lengthwise in half and cut each half into three pieces.
3. Marinate the potatoes in the lemon mixture for 30 minutes or more.
4. Preheat the oven to 190°C/375°F/Gas mark 5.
5. Place the dish in the hot oven and cook for 40 minutes. About 20 minutes before the end, turn the potatoes over.
6. Sprinkle with salt before serving.

## Ingredient Info: Saffron

Read about saffron on page 63.

# Spinach in Clarified Butter

**This is the simplest and healthiest way of cooking spinach, as it ensures most of the nutrients are retained**

| | | | |
|---|---|---|---|
| O | suitable | B | suitable |
| A | omit the pepper | AB | omit the pepper |

SERVES 4

2lb/1kg spinach, stems trimmed
3 tbsp clarified butter (see recipe page 187)

Sea salt and freshly ground black pepper

1. Rinse the spinach several times and spin or dry it to get rid of the water.
2. Heat the clarified butter in a large pan or wok and add the spinach. With two wooden spoons stir the spinach until it wilts. This should take 5 minutes. Add salt and freshly ground black pepper. Serve.

## Ingredient Info: Spinach

Read about spinach in Spinach with Currants and Pine Nuts (page 94) and Spinach Salad with Walnut Oil (page 75).

# Spinach with Currants and Pine Nuts

This way of cooking spinach comes from a traditional Catalan recipe, but similar preparations are also found in other countries around the Mediterranean.

O    suitable

A    omit the pepper

B    choose the pine nuts

AB   choose the pine nuts and omit the pepper

SERVES 4

---

2lb/1kg spinach, stems trimmed

3 tbsp clarified butter (see recipe page 187)

2 tbsp currants

Sea salt and freshly ground black pepper

2 tbsp roasted pine nuts or hazelnuts (see page 194)

1.  Rinse the spinach several times and spin or dry it to get rid of the water.
2.  Heat the clarified butter in a large pan or wok and add the spinach. With two wooden spoons stir the spinach until it wilts. This should take 5 minutes. During this time add the currants. Add salt and freshly ground black pepper.
3.  Sprinkle the roasted nuts over the spinach before serving.

## Ingredient Info: Spinach

Spinach contains more than double the amount of carotenoids found in carrots. It also is a very rich source of chlorophyll, a green plant pigment that has potent anti-cancer properties and is very cleansing to the body. Avoid overcooking spinach as this destroys some of its goodness. Eat fresh spinach as often as you possibly can. Studies have shown it to be the vegetable most often eaten by those who are most protected against cancer.

Read more about spinach on page 75.

# Stuffed Courgette Flowers

Those of you who are lucky enough to have vegetable gardens can enjoy this easy, colourful and delicious recipe. The season for courgette (zucchini) flowers is late spring, summer and early autumn.

O   suitable                           B   suitable
A   omit the pepper                    AB  omit the pepper

SERVES 4

| | |
|---|---|
| 12 courgette (zucchini) flowers | Sea salt and freshly ground black pepper |
| ½lb/225g fresh goat's cheese | 1 garlic clove, crushed |
| Olive oil | 1 tsp thyme, preferably fresh |

1.  Place the cheese and a little olive oil in a mixing bowl and mash together lightly. Add salt and pepper to taste.
2.  Divide the cheese mixture between two bowls. Add the crushed garlic to one bowl and the thyme to the other.
3.  Remove the stamens from the flowers. Form six elongated olives with each mixture and delicately stuff the flowers.
4.  Lightly heat the flowers in olive oil until the cheese has softened. Serve immediately.

# Stuffed Courgettes

**Stuffed courgettes (zucchinis) make an excellent appetizer, or are particularly good as an accompaniment to lamb chops. Round courgettes are great for stuffing, so use these whenever they're available.**

O  suitable

A  not suitable

B  not suitable

AB  omit the pepper

SERVES 4

| | |
|---|---|
| 4 small round courgettes (zucchinis) or | 1 handful of raisins |
|     4 short plump ones | 2 tbsp pine nuts, optional |
| 4 medium shallots, finely chopped | Sea salt and freshly ground black pepper |
| Olive oil | 4 tomatoes |
| 1 tbsp thyme, preferably fresh | 4 garlic cloves, crushed |
| 3 slices of spelt bread | |

1. Preheat the oven to 150°C/300°F/Gas mark 2.
2. Sauté the shallots in a little olive oil until they soften. Add the thyme and set aside.
3. During this time soak the bread in lukewarm water, then squeeze out the liquid.
4. If you're using round courgettes (zucchinis), cut the "hats" off the top and scoop out the insides. For long courgettes (zucchinis), cut them in two lengthwise and scoop out the flesh to give a canoe shape. Take care not to break through the outer skin. Cook the chopped insides of the courgettes (zucchinis) in the olive oil. Set aside.
5. Roast the pine nuts (see Basic Recipes page 194).
6. Mix together the shallots, bread, cooked courgette (zucchini) flesh, pine nuts, raisins, salt and pepper, and stuff the courgette (zucchini) shells with the mixture.
7. Soak the tomatoes in boiling water for 30 seconds, then peel them. Discard the seeds and juice and finely chop the tomatoes.
8. Place the chopped tomatoes and crushed garlic at the bottom of a shallow earthenware dish.
9. Arrange the stuffed courgettes (zucchinis) on the tomato mixture and bake in the oven for 1 hour.

# Vegetables in Olive Oil

**This warming and comforting dish is good during the winter months.**

O  not suitable

A  suitable

B  suitable

AB  suitable

SERVES 4–6

8–12 medium carrots, cut into 3

8–12 little white and purple turnips, scrubbed not
   peeled

8–12 small onions

12–16 shallots

16–24 garlic cloves, unpeeled

3 fennel bulbs, quartered

2 tbsp olive oil

20–30 chestnuts, already cooked or vacuum
   packed

Salt to taste

1.  Steam the vegetables in the following order. Start with the carrots. Five
    minutes later add the turnips, onions, shallots and garlic. Keep an eye on the
    cooking and after another 5 minutes add the fennel. Cook for a further 10
    minutes. The vegetables should be just tender.
2.  Heat the olive oil in a frying pan (skillet) and sauté the vegetables with the
    chestnuts for a few minutes. Shake the pan so that nothing sticks to the bottom.
    The vegetables should be golden in places; this step enhances the flavour.
    Season to taste.

# Vegetables with Rosemary

**The secret to this recipe is in the cutting.**

O   suitable

A   omit the pepper

B   suitable

AB  omit the pepper

SERVES 4

1 tbsp olive oil

4 large garlic cloves, cut into thick slices

6 medium carrots, cut at a slant

4 tbsp fresh rosemary leaves

2 fennel bulbs, cut into 8 or 12 according to size

2 courgettes (zucchinis), cut into 8 or 12

Sea salt and freshly ground black pepper

1. Heat the olive oil in a large frying pan (skillet) or wok. Add the garlic, then the carrots and rosemary and let this cook a few minutes, stirring constantly. Add enough water just to cover the bottom of the pan and cook for 15 minutes. Check on the water and add more if necessary to prevent the carrots burning.
2. Add the fennel and let it cook 10 minutes, watching the water level all the time.
3. Finally add the courgettes (zucchinis) and cook for a few minutes. The vegetables should be barely cooked. Season and serve.

# Wild Rice

Wild rice can be served with meat, game or salad. It can be used as the base for a stuffing or you can stir fry it with mushrooms, onions, celery, herbs etc.

| | | | | |
|---|---|---|---|---|
| O | suitable | | B | not suitable |
| A | suitable | | AB | suitable |

SERVES 4—6

---

1 cup/200g wild rice
2¼ cups/500ml cold water

¾ tsp sea salt

1. Wash the wild rice thoroughly before cooking and discard the rinsing water.
2. Place the rice, water and salt in a heavy saucepan with a solid lid. Cover, bring to the boil, then immediately reduce the heat. Simmer for 45–60 minutes or until most of the kernels have opened, but are still fairly chewy. Fluff with a fork.

Cooking times will vary for wild rice from different origins so it's vital to keep an eye on the process. Check the rice after 30 minutes. If there is not enough water at the bottom of the pan, add more boiling water. If it is cooked and water remains, pour off the excess. Be sure not to overcook the wild rice as it will become mushy.

## Variation

To add aroma to the wild rice, cook in a herbal infusion. Boil 2¼ cups/500ml water, add 1 teaspoon of thyme, rosemary and savory. Leave to steep for 10 minutes then drain through a sieve. Cook the rice in this liquid.

## Ingredient Info: Wild rice

Wild rice is not only a gourmet's treat but is also highly nutritious. It contains more protein than most cereals, is low in fat and rich in the minerals which have been lost in polished white rice.

# Courgette Flower Fritters

**Ensure your flowers are as fresh as possible, as they only last for a short time after being picked. This is made easier if you have your own vegetable garden or if you know of someone who grows courgettes (zucchinis).**

O   suitable

A   suitable

B   use cow's milk

AB   suitable

SERVES 4

12 courgette (zucchini) flowers with their little
     courgettes (zucchinis) attached

1 organic egg

2 tbsp spelt flour

4 tbsp soya milk

3 tbsp olive oil

Sea salt

1.  In a bowl, whip the egg, flour and milk for the batter. Set aside.
2.  Heat the olive oil in a frying pan (skillet) – it must not smoke.
3.  Plunge the flowers with their courgettes (zucchinis) in the batter and gently fry 5 minutes on each side.
4.  Sprinkle with salt and serve immediately.

# Courgette Purée

**Choose organic courgettes (zucchinis) as they contain less water and will make your purée less liquid.**

O   suitable

A   suitable

B   suitable

AB   suitable

SERVES 4

2lb/1kg courgettes (zucchinis), cut into slices

Extra virgin olive oil

2 garlic cloves, crushed

6–8 large leaves fresh sweet basil

Sea salt

Freshly ground black pepper, optional

1.  Steam the courgettes (zucchinis) for 10 minutes.
2.  Blend the courgettes (zucchinis) in a food processor with the olive oil, crushed garlic, sweet basil, salt and pepper.

# goat's cheese

Goat's cheese is becoming increasingly popular as more and more people realize that not only does it taste wonderful, but for many it is easier to digest than traditional cow's milk cheeses. Humans tolerate goat's milk better than cow's milk because the biological characteristics of the curd and fat in goat's milk make it easier to digest. In addition, its protein content and amino acid composition is close to human milk. For this reason it has been used traditionally in infant feeding to replace cow's milk.

There is now a burgeoning number of goat's cheese makers who are producing a wonderfully diverse range of cheeses, each with its own characteristic taste. Many of the cheeses are still made on small farms and these are among the most interesting. And don't forget that goat's cheese isn't just for spreading, it also adds a distinctive flavour to cooked dishes.

# Crêpes with Goat's Cheese and Green Sauce

**This recipe makes 12 crêpes. When making the batter, use the type of milk most suited to your blood type.**

O  suitable

A  omit the pepper

B  suitable

AB  omit the pepper

SERVES 4

---

3 organic eggs

6 tbsp spelt flour

¾ cup/200ml milk: soya, goat or cow

1 pinch sea salt

Olive oil or clarified butter (see recipe page 187)
  for the pan

3 fresh goat's cheeses

Freshly ground black pepper

Fresh Coriander or Basil Sauce (see recipes
  pages 139 and 143)

1.  Beat the eggs in a mixing bowl, then incorporate the flour, milk and salt to form a dough. If you have the time let the dough sit for 2 hours, otherwise proceed.
2.  Heat a small amount of oil or clarified butter in a non-stick frying pan (skillet). Pour in enough batter to make a crêpe. Flip it over when the first side is done.
3.  Cover one half of the crêpe with some finely sliced goat's cheese. Fold over the other half and continue cooking until the cheese is melted. Sprinkle with freshly ground black pepper. Serve as you make them or keep them warm in a slow oven.
4.  Spread each crêpe with 3 teaspoons of coriander or basil sauce.

# Goat's Cheese Dumplings

O   suitable

A   omit the pepper

B   omit the sesame seeds

AB  omit the sesame seeds and pepper

SERVES 4

---

1lb/450g soft mild fresh goat's cheese

4 organic eggs

6–8 tbsp spelt flour

1 tsp sea salt

2 tbsp roasted sesame seeds (see guidance page
    194), optional

Olive oil

SAUCE:

10oz/300g soya yogurt, goat's milk yogurt or
    natural yogurt

2 tbsp chopped fresh chives or dill

½ garlic clove

1 tbsp extra virgin olive oil

Sea salt and freshly ground black pepper

1. If your cheese is too moist, remove some whey by draining it through a cloth in a colander. The drier the cheese the better. Mix the eggs one by one into the cheese. Add the flour, starting with 6 tablespoons and increasing to 8 tablespoons if necessary, then the salt. The texture should be like a light dough. If the mixture is too runny you will need more flour – this depends on the humidity of the cheese and the size of the eggs.
2. On a floured surface roll a fifth of the dough into a 1 inch/2.5cm wide sausage. Cut the sausage into 1¼ inch/3cm segments of dough, and lightly flour both sides of each dumpling.
3. Fill a large saucepan with salted water and bring to the boil. Slowly drop 10–15 dumplings into the water. When they resurface they are cooked. Remove from the water with a slotted spoon and place on a dry dish towel. If some dumplings stick to the bottom of the pan carefully release them and they will float up to the surface. Do likewise with the rest of the dough.
4. Mix all the sauce ingredients together and check the seasoning.
5. Lightly brown the dumplings in olive oil. Serve them sprinkled with grilled sesame seeds, and accompanied by the sauce.

# Goat's Cheese with Tarragon and Shallots

**This is an excellent recipe for those who like salty things at breakfast time. Try serving the cheese on rye or spelt bread, or you may also spread it on chicory leaves and celery stalks for lunch.**

O   suitable

A   omit the pepper

B   suitable

AB  omit the pepper

---

½lb/225g soft mild fresh goat's cheese

3 tbsp finely chopped fresh tarragon

3 tbsp olive oil

2oz/50g shallots, finely chopped

Sea salt and freshly ground black pepper, optional

1.  Mix all the ingredients together. Set aside in a cool place for an hour, or better still several hours, for all the aromas to blend.

## Ingredient Info: Tarragon

Read about this herb on page 64.

# snails

Snails contain a beneficial lectin capable of agglutinating mutated A-like cancer cells, especially breast cancer cells. They are therefore highly beneficial for As and ABs. This surprising discovery about snails was made by Dr Peter D'Adamo during his research. "The edible snail, *Helix pomatia*, is a powerful breast cancer agglutinin capable of determining whether the cancerous cells will metastasize to the lymph nodes."

While we were doing our cooking sessions in the Touraine in France we visited an organic snail farm owned by a very knowledgeable "white collar" businessman who had redirected his energy into raising snails. He told us the story of a 70-year-old woman he had recently met whose uncle had a snail farm in Switzerland during the last world war. She spent some time with him and over a period of three months he cured her asthma simply by giving her snail broth.

Snails are widely available in France but are harder to find in the UK and US. However, if you do manage to obtain them, try these recipes – you'll be pleasantly surprised at just how tasty snails are. And don't forget to look for them on the menu next time you visit a French restaurant. Type Bs are the only ones who should avoid snails.

# Snails with Oregano and Shallots

**Serve the snails on their own or on a slice of spelt toast rubbed with a garlic clove.**

O   suitable

A   suitable

B   not suitable

AB  suitable

SERVES 4

---

10 shallots, finely sliced

4 garlic cloves

2 tbsp olive oil

1 tbsp fresh oregano

¾lb/350g snails, canned or vacuum packed
  (cooked in a court-bouillon)

1 large bunch of flat-leaf parsley, finely chopped

1.  Lightly brown the shallots and garlic in the olive oil.
2.  Add the oregano when the shallots are slightly golden and simmer until the shallots are soft. Add the snails and heat until they are piping hot – about 5 minutes.
3.  Just before serving, add the parsley.

# Snails in a Green Sauce

**Snails are a traditional food in France. Years ago when housewives had the time or if the family had a cook, snails were gathered after rainy days. They are most often served with a garlic and parsley butter. You can find them in some delicatessens already cooked and preserved either in a jar, a can or vacuum packed. All you need to do is reheat them and serve with an accompanying sauce. When buying snails, look out for the word _helix_ on the label. If they come from Asia they may have used another animal called Achatine. This is not a real snail.**

O   suitable

A   suitable

B   not suitable

AB  suitable

SERVES 4

---

¾lb/350g snails, canned or vacuum packed
  (cooked in a court-bouillon)

Fresh Coriander or Sweet Basil Sauce (see
  recipes on pages 139 and 143)

1.  Steam the snails for about 8–10 minutes and just before serving mix them with the sauce of your choice. Serve on spelt or rye toast.

# seafood

Eating a portion of fish twice a week can cut your risk of coronary artery disease in half. This was the result of a 20-year study that took place in the Netherlands and was published in 1985 in the *New England Journal of Medicine*. The omega 3 fatty acids present in cold water fish such as mackerel, herring, sardines, salmon, tuna and trout are precursors to short-lived hormone-like substances called prostaglandins that can inhibit blood clotting and counter inflammatory responses. In addition, the type of fat in these cold water fish has anti-inflammatory effects that have been shown to relieve asthma, arthritis, psoriasis and eczema. The protein in fish also has a beneficial effect on brain neurotransmitters, boosting mental energy.

All blood types should include fish as part of their weekly diet, though do check in the food lists which fish are suitable. Despite polluted oceans, wild fish are still preferable to farmed fish. Wild fish eat the same food they have been finding for millions of years, whereas some farm-reared fish are fed with grain and treated with antibiotics – not exactly their natural choice. Also, the space they have to live in is restricted and this increases their risk of illness. Farm-reared salmon has more fat under its skin and the quality of the oils is not that of the wild fish. Although higher in fat, they have very little omega-3 oil. This information is not to discourage you from eating fish but rather to encourage you to make the best possible choice.

Choose your fish according to the season. Your fishmonger will help you out with this and will tell you whether the fish is wild or not. Avoid overcooking as this will reduce the health benefits and dry out the flesh. Also avoid aluminium foil, as this metal can very easily become toxic in your body if it is present in excessive amounts. Use greaseproof (waxed) paper instead. Cooking methods should retain the nutrient-rich juices. Poaching (don't forget to use the cooking liquid) and light grilling (broiling) are preferred ways of cooking fish. Many people like to steam fish, but with this method most of the valuable fish juices fall into the cooking water and are thrown away.

# Baked Fish with Shallots and Ginger

| O | suitable | B | suitable |
|---|----------|---|----------|
| A | suitable | AB | suitable |

SERVES 4

4 fillets (1⅓lb/600g) white fish such as cod

2 tbsp olive oil

¾ cup/100g shallots, finely chopped

1 tbsp fresh ginger root, finely grated

Sea salt

Juice of 1 lemon

1. Preheat the oven 190°C/375°F/Gas mark 5.
2. Use a little of the olive oil to oil an ovenware dish big enough to take the four fillets.
3. Sprinkle three-quarters of the chopped shallots over the bottom of the dish. Place the fish on top of the shallots.
4. Cover the fish with the remaining shallots, add the grated ginger root and a sprinkling of salt.
5. Drizzle the remaining oil over the fish and pour the lemon juice around the fish.
6. Bake in the oven for around 20 minutes.

## Ingredient Info: Ginger root

See information on Three Ginger Cake page 171 and Green Tea with Ginger page 161.

# Cod Steaks in Yogurt and Spices

**For this recipe we were inspired by Indian cuisine. When you cook with yogurt you will find the sauce has a tendency to separate, leaving a creamy part and a watery part – this is normal.**

O   suitable

A   omit the pepper

B   suitable

AB   omit the pepper

SERVES 4

| | |
|---|---|
| 4 cod steaks, ½lb/225g each | I tsp sea salt |
| I tsp cumin seeds, roasted | I tbsp clarified butter (see recipe page 187) |
| 1½ cups/340ml sheep's yogurt | 4 medium onions, cut into thin slices |
| 2 garlic cloves, crushed | Freshly ground black pepper |
| I tsp turmeric | 2 tbsp chopped fresh coriander (cilantro) |
| I tsp grated fresh ginger root | I lime, cut into 4 segments |

1. Preheat the oven to 190°C/350°F/Gas mark 5.
2. In a mortar grind the roasted cumin seeds. Add the yogurt, crushed garlic, turmeric, grated ginger and salt.
3. In a large pan melt the clarified butter and cook the onions for 5 minutes until they become translucent.
4. Spread the onions on the bottom of an ovenware dish large enough to hold the four pieces of fish. Spoon 3 tablespoons of the yogurt sauce over the onions, place the fish on the onions and cover the fish with the rest of the sauce.
5. Bake in the oven for 40 minutes.
6. Grind some pepper over the fish, sprinkle with fresh coriander (cilantro) and serve with the lime segments.

## Ingredient Info: Cumin

Read about cumin seeds in the Cucumber Raita recipe on page 66.

## Ingredient Info: Turmeric

Turmeric is a well known remedy in Ayurveda – an ancient Indian health system. Traditionally it is used for intestinal disorders such as diarrhoea, flatulence, worms, gastritis, acidity and nausea. It is also recommended for jaundice, skin conditions such as psoriasis, fungal infections, boils and ringworm. Generally it is used as an antiseptic. Research has been looking at the properties of turmeric for several decades and has confirmed the value of these traditional uses.

The active ingredient in turmeric – curcumin – has marked antioxidant and anti-inflammatory effects, making it a good remedy (taken in capsule form) for rheumatoid arthritis, asthma and eczema. In one study curcumin was shown to be as effective as cortisone in acute inflammation. Turmeric also benefits the liver, by increasing bile secretion and solubility.

Turmeric has been shown to have cancer-protective effects in animal studies and research is underway to discover if this translates to humans. Although more human studies are needed to evaluate the role turmeric could play in the prevention of cancer, it seems reasonable to recommend that turmeric be included in a cancer-prevention program. As and ABs should include turmeric in their diet and add it to their choice of supplements.

# Gravlax

**Marinated wild salmon is delicious and what could be more satisfying than making one's own Gravlax in the summer.**

O   suitable
A   use the black mustard seeds

B   suitable
AB   use the black mustard seeds

SERVES 6–8

---

1 wild salmon, approx. 3lbs/1.5 kg
1 tbsp black peppercorns or black mustard seeds,
    crushed
4–5 tbsp sea salt, coarsely ground
4–5 tbsp brown sugar
2 cups/500ml fresh dill, finely chopped

GRAVLAX SAUCE:
1 tbsp lemon juice
2 tbsp brown sugar
6 tbsp vinegar-free Dijon style mustard
⅔ cup/140ml olive oil
4 tbsp finely chopped fresh dill

1. Ask your fishmonger to scale, bone and fillet the salmon, leaving on the skin. At home pull out any remaining bones – a pair of tweezers will come in handy.
2. Using a mortar lightly crush the peppercorns or mustard seeds and mix with the sea salt, sugar and dill. In a non-metallic dish lay one of the fillets skin-side down. Cover with the salt-sugar-dill mixture. Lay the remaining fillet, skin-side up, on top of the first fillet.
3. Place a plate the size of the dish on the fish and cover with cling film. Place a heavy weight (stones, jars of honey etc.) on the plate.
4. Allow it to marinate in the refrigerator for 48 hours. Turn the 2 fillets over, without separating them, every 12 hours.
5. When you are nearly ready to serve the fish, make the sauce. Mix the lemon juice, sugar and mustard. Slowly add the olive oil, drop by drop, stirring constantly. The sauce will thicken like a mayonnaise. Just before serving stir in the dill.
6. When ready to serve, place the fillets, skin-side down, on the cutting board. Scrape off the pepper or mustard seeds and dill. Cut slices, beginning at the tail end, without cutting through the skin. A special salmon knife or a long, thin-bladed knife will make the cutting easier.
7. Serve with its sauce, lemon slices and thinly sliced toasted spelt or rye bread and butter.

## Ingredient Info: Salmon

This is perhaps the best way to eat salmon. When fish is raw, you get the most benefit from the omega-3 fatty acids.

# Grilled Tuna

**We have discovered how delicious fresh tuna fish can be when you barely cook it. Tuna can become dry very quickly. This way it remains moist inside.**

O  suitable                   B  suitable
A  suitable                   AB suitable

SERVES 4

2 slices of tuna fish weighing
   1¼–1½lb/560g–675g

1. Preheat the grill (broiler) until it is hot enough so that the fish is "seized" and the juices retained. For a 1¼ inch/3cm slice, grill (broil) the fish 5 minutes on the first side and 2 minutes on the other side.
2. If you prefer bite-size pieces, cut the slices in 1¼ inch/3cm cubes and grill (broil) on both sides but be sure to keep an eye on the cooking – the fish must not be over cooked.
3. We serve the tuna with one of our sauces – take your pick from Soya Yogurt Dill Sauce on page 142, Ginger and Tamari Sauce on page 140, Sweet Basil Sauce on page 143 or Fresh Coriander (cilantro) Sauce on page 139.

## Ingredient Info: Tuna

Tuna is one of the few fish high in omega-3 fatty acids. Wild salmon, mackerel, sardines and trout are in the same category.

# Marinated Grilled Tuna

O   suitable

A   suitable

B   suitable

AB  suitable

SERVES 4

1½lb/675g tuna, cut into 1 inch/2.5cm thick slices

MARINADE:

5 tbsp lemon juice

5 tbsp olive oil

1 tbsp finely chopped fresh sweet basil – in the winter use fresh rosemary

1. Mix the marinade ingredients together. Coat both sides of the fish slices with the marinade and leave for several hours in a covered container in the refrigerator.

2. Cook the fish either under a grill (broiler) or in a frying pan (skillet). The grilling should sear the outside of the fish and leave it practically raw inside – 5 minutes on one side and 2 minutes on the other should be enough.

# Monkfish en Papillote

**This fish will render a fair amount of natural juices. Be sure to enjoy them.**

| | | | |
|---|---|---|---|
| O | suitable | B | suitable |
| A | suitable | AB | suitable |

SERVES 4

1¾lb/780g monkfish, cut into 4 pieces
1 tbsp olive oil
1 tsp freshly squeezed lemon juice

Fresh Coriander (cilantro) or Parsley Sauce to
serve (pages 139 and 141)

1. Preheat the oven to 180°C/350°F/Gas mark 4.
2. Marinate the fish fillets in the olive oil and lemon juice for 10 minutes.
3. Cut 4 large pieces of greaseproof (waxed) paper into 30 x 30cm/12 x 12 inch squares.
4. Place each fillet in the middle of a square. Gather the 4 corners tightly around the fish and tie.
5. The fish must cook slowly in its own juices. Bake in the preheated oven for 20 minutes.
6. Serve the fish packages immediately, accompanied by either of the green sauces. (We do not salt the fish as the sauce has sufficient salt.)

# Salmon Mousse

**Summer, when wild salmon is in season, is the best time to make this dish. If you are expecting guests you can prepare it a day in advance.**

| O | suitable | B | suitable |
|---|----------|---|----------|
| A | omit the pepper | AB | omit the pepper |

SERVES 6–8

---

1½lb/675g fresh salmon, preferably wild

2 shallots, roughly chopped

2 celery stalks, roughly chopped

3 carrots, peeled and roughly chopped

4 tbsp chopped fresh parsley

1 bunch dill, chopped

½ cup/125ml Mayonnaise (see recipe page 190)

3 tsp sea salt

Freshly ground black pepper

6 tbsp agar agar

3 tbsp lemon juice

⅔ cup/140ml fish court bouillon from salmon

Fresh dill and parsley to garnish

COURT BOUILLON:

2 onions

2 celery stalks

4 parsley sprigs

1 bay leaf

1 tsp fresh thyme

1 tsp sea salt

1. Line a 1.1 litre pudding basin (5 cup mould) with greaseproof (waxed) paper.
2. Put the ingredients for the court bouillon into a large saucepan, cover with cold water, add the salmon and heat to simmering point. Simmer for 15 minutes, then allow the fish to cool in the liquid.
3. Put the cold fish in a colander to let any excess liquid drain off. Set aside ⅔ cup/140ml of the court bouillon.
4. Break up the salmon, removing skin and bones. Place in the food processor bowl and process. Add the roughly chopped vegetables, parsley and dill. Pulse the ingredients until smooth, but leaving some visible particles of vegetable. Place in a large mixing bowl.
5. Add the mayonnaise, salt and pepper.
6. Melt the agar agar in the lemon juice, add the court bouillon and bring to the boil. Stir until dissolved. Pour this mixture into the processed fish and vegetables. Stir well. Adjust the seasoning if necessary. Spoon into the basin (mould), cover and refrigerate overnight.
7. Before serving, remove from the basin (mould) onto a serving platter, and garnish with dill and parsley.

# Salmon, Lime and Dill Tartare

**Make this delicious tartare in summer, when wild salmon is available. It is less fatty than farmed salmon and its valuable fatty acids, taste and texture are far superior.**

O    suitable

A    omit black pepper

B    suitable

AB   omit black pepper

SERVES 4

---

1½lb/675g wild salmon

Zest and juice of 1 non-treated lime

½ bunch fresh dill, finely chopped

Sea salt and freshly ground black pepper

Lettuce leaves for serving

1. Using a boning knife, remove the skin and bones from the salmon.
2. While you are working, keep the fish as fresh as possible. Place some ice cubes in a large bowl, then place a smaller bowl inside the first one. Chop the salmon into tiny pieces with a very sharp knife, and place each piece in the chilled bowl. Do not use a food processor as this produces a sticky consistency.
3. Add the lime juice, zest, dill, salt and pepper.
4. Taste and adjust seasoning if necessary. Serve chilled on lettuce leaves.

# Wild Sea Bass

**Perhaps the finest of all fish, bass is at its best wild. This is another fish that is often farm raised. Do your best to find the one that has grown up in the wild blue seas.**

O    suitable

A    suitable

B    not suitable

AB   not suitable

SERVES 4

---

4 × 1lb/450g wild sea bass, scaled and gutted
    (cleaned)
4 tsp fennel seeds
Sea salt and freshly ground black pepper

DRESSING:
3 tbsp extra virgin olive oil
Juice of 1 lemon
Finely chopped fresh chives
Sea salt

1.  Sprinkle the fish inside and out with the fennel seeds, salt and pepper.
2.  Steam the fish for 20 minutes until they are no longer pink inside. This cooking method allows one to appreciate the fine and flavourful meat of the bass.
3.  Mix together the olive oil, lemon juice, chives and salt to make the sauce. Ordinary olive oil can have a slightly acidic taste. The best varieties are fruity, highly aromatic and don't have that initial bite on the tongue.
4.  Serve the fish with its dressing.

# meat, poultry and game

Wild animals are what our very first ancestors hunted and fed themselves with. An animal which has matured in the wilderness (some game is reared on farms; it is therefore still "game" but no longer wild) has the highest quality meat. It is the most natural and therefore best for your health. These animals eat wild plants that have not been altered by man; they live in the outdoors, benefiting from the fresh air and sunshine; and they live their own natural life.

Factory-farmed animals, in contrast, live in confined areas; are fed pesticide-, herbicide- and fungicide-treated grains; are injected with hormones and given antibiotics. The hormones fatten the animals up quickly, while the antibiotics are necessary to fight the frequent infections that result from cramped conditions.

Organic domesticated animals that are reared outdoors in natural pastures, and that are treated and killed with respect, are a much better food. And if you're not convinced by the animal welfare argument, do bear in mind that there is also the question of quality. Wild and respectfully-reared animals seem to have more essential fats and less fat in the meaty parts.

Chicken is another highly tampered-with food product. Mass production methods use hormones, antibiotics and feed that is grown with the aid of pesticides – these are all substances you absorb when you eat the meat. Some battery-raised chickens live in such tightly-packed conditions that the feathers on their backs are worn away. Taste a chicken that is raised on a farm where it sees the sunshine and eats the worms from the earth. Compare it to a battery-raised chicken and you will not want to turn back.

# Braised Beef

This is a festive dish for close friends and family on a cold winter's day. Cook the meat the day before so that you can remove the fat. This enables easier cutting and neater slices. If you've never tried marrow, do give it a go. For the vegetables we used the freshest seasonal ones, so make your choice from whatever is at its prime.

| | | | |
|---|---|---|---|
| O | suitable | B | suitable |
| A | not suitable | AB | not suitable |

SERVES 4

---

3lb/1.5kg fully trimmed bottom or top round of beef for braising

4 marrow bones, optional

4 tbsp olive oil

1lb/450g onions, finely sliced

1 2 cups/250–500ml stock or water

1 bay leaf

Coarse sea salt

20 black peppercorns

1lb/450g carrots

1lb/450g little turnips

1lb/450g onions

2 courgettes (zucchinis)

TO SERVE:

Dijon mustard, preferably with mustard seeds

Fresh Coriander Sauce (see recipe page 139)

Aïoli (see recipe page 138)

Hot spelt toast for the marrow, optional

1. Preheat the oven to 150°C/300°F/Gas mark 2.
2. Place the olive oil in a cast iron casserole, add the onions and sauté them until they become golden. Move the onions to the side of the casserole, add the meat and brown it on all sides. Add enough stock or water to cover the onions, and add the bay leaf, salt and peppercorns. Transfer the casserole to the oven and cook for 3 hours. Check the amount of liquid at the bottom of the casserole and add more if necessary.
3. Let the meat cool off in the casserole, then put the casserole in the refrigerator overnight. The next morning, remove the fat that has risen to the top by scraping it off with a spoon.
4. Steam the vegetables starting with those needing the longest cooking time: the carrots, then the turnips, followed by the onions and courgettes (zucchinis).
5. At the same time slowly heat the meat for 20–30 minutes in its juices (with the marrow bones, if using).
6. Serve the meat topped with the thickened onion sauce, and accompanied by the marrow bones and the steamed vegetables.
7. Place on the table the aïoli, the fresh coriander sauce, the mustard, coarse sea salt, the pepper grinder and hot toast.

# Braised Lamb with Onions and Lemons

**Lamb is an excellent meat for blood types O and B. ABs can also eat lamb but in smaller quantities. The lemon in this dish gives a tangy contrast to the very characteristic flavour of the lamb.**

| O | suitable | B | suitable |
|---|----------|---|----------|
| A | not suitable | AB | omit the pepper |

SERVES 4

---

3lb/1.5kg neck of lamb with bones

2 tbsp olive oil

2lb/1kg finely sliced onions

1 cup/250ml water

Fine sea salt and freshly ground black pepper

1 tbsp thyme (fresh or dried)

1 non-treated lemon, cut into slices then halved

Zest of 1 non-treated lemon

Freshly chopped coriander (cilantro) leaves

1. Trim any excess fat from the meat. In a cast iron casserole, brown the meat on all sides in 1 tablespoon of olive oil. Remove the meat and set aside.
2. Add the remaining oil to the casserole and cook the onions until they become translucent. Now add the water.
3. Place the meat on the onions, add the salt, pepper, thyme and halved lemon slices. Cover and simmer for 1½ hours. Be sure to maintain enough liquid at the bottom of the casserole. If necessary add more water.
4. During this time prepare the lemon zest. If you have a special peeler use it, if not use a vegetable peeler. Cut the lemon zest into neat julienne strips. Drop in boiling water for 3 minutes, then drain.
5. Before serving the lamb, sprinkle with the lemon zest and fresh coriander (cilantro).

# Marinated Shoulder of Lamb

**A leg of lamb could also be used in this recipe.**

O  suitable

A  not suitable

B  suitable

AB  omit the pepper

SERVES 4–6

2½–3lb/1.2–1.4 kg shoulder of lamb

MARINADE:

10 garlic cloves, roughly chopped

2 sprigs sage

3 sprigs rosemary

3 tbsp olive oil

Juice of 1 lemon

Sea salt and freshly ground black pepper

1.  The night before, or at least 4 hours in advance, mix the marinade ingredients together and coat both sides of the meat with the mixture. Cover the meat and from time to time turn it over so that all the aromas can penetrate the meat.
2.  Preheat the oven to 200°C/400°F/Gas mark 6.
3.  Season the meat with salt and freshly ground black pepper, place on a roasting pan and roast for 30–45 minutes, depending on how well done you like your meat. Halfway through the cooking, turn the meat over.
4.  Remove the meat from the oven, cover it and let it sit for 10–15 minutes before carving. This allows the juices to settle in the meat and prevents so much of the juice being lost during carving.

# Our Osso Buco

Osso Buco is an Italian dish of veal shanks. Our version is easy to prepare and has a zesty flavouring. It can be cooked in the morning for serving in the evening as it improves by being reheated.

| | | | |
|---|---|---|---|
| O | use stock or water | B | suitable |
| A | not suitable | AB | not suitable |

SERVES 4

4 x 1¼ inch/3cm veal shank slices
2lb/1kg finely sliced onions
4 tbsp olive oil or butter
20 sage leaves
1 pinch fine sea salt
Freshly ground pepper
1 cup/250ml dry white wine, water or stock

GREMOLATA:
8–10 walnuts
4 tbsp fresh flat-leaf parsley, finely chopped
2 garlic cloves, finely chopped
Grated zest of 2 non-treated lemons

1. Preheat the oven to 150°C/300°F/Gas mark 2.
2. Place half the oil or butter in a heavy cast iron casserole large enough for the 4 slices of veal not to overlap. Add the meat and brown on both sides. Remove the meat and set aside.
3. In the same casserole, brown the sliced onions in the rest of the oil or butter. Add the sage leaves.
4. Remove half the onions. Place the meat on the bed of onions in the casserole, sprinkle with salt and pepper, and cover with the remaining onions.
5. Pour the liquid over the meat and onions, cover the casserole and place in the oven for 2 hours. Every half hour check the liquid and add more if necessary.
6. While the meat is cooking, prepare the gremolata. Shell the walnuts and grill them (see instructions page 194), chop and mix with the parsley, garlic and lemon zests.
7. When ready to serve, remove the meat and blend the onions with a hand-held blender in the casserole. You may also leave them as they are. Adjust the seasoning if necessary.
8. Serve the onions with the meat, and place the gremolata in a serving dish for diners to sprinkle it over as they wish.

# Steak Tartare

If you've never eaten raw beef (apart from the pink bit in the middle of your steak) do give it a try – it's delicious and has more enzymes than cooked meat. Serve with a green salad and, if your blood type allows, our Oven Fries (see page 90). Steak tartare is usually made with a raw yolk of egg. We prefer mayonnaise, which gives a rich velvety consistency.

O   suitable                          B    suitable
A   not suitable                      AB  not suitable

SERVES 4

---

1½lb/675g lean beef, freshly ground          4 tbsp flat-leaf parsley, finely chopped
5–7 tbsp Mayonnaise (see page 190)           8 large basil leaves, cut in thin strips with scissors
2 garlic cloves, finely crushed              1–2 tsp cider vinegar
8 green onions, finely chopped               Sea salt and freshly ground black pepper
3 tbsp chives, finely chopped

1.  Place all the ingredients in a large bowl and mix thoroughly.
2.  Taste and adjust the seasoning if necessary. Serve immediately or refrigerate until serving time.

## Ingredient Info: Raw meat

Raw meat is packed with goodness – if it's best quality, organic and fresh. If you are worried about parasites in meat you can freeze it for 14 days prior to eating.

# Chicken with Preserved Lemons

**Saffron and preserved lemons give this chicken dish an oriental touch.**

O   suitable

A   omit the pepper

B   not suitable

AB  not suitable

SERVES 4

---

3–4lb/1.3–1.8kg free-range chicken, cut into 12 pieces

3 large onions

2 tbsp olive oil

1 tbsp ground ginger

Sea salt and freshly ground black pepper

1 cup/250ml water or Chicken Stock (see recipe page 184)

1 pinch saffron strands, lightly crushed

1–2 Preserved Lemons (see page 191), peel only

1 bunch fresh coriander (cilantro)

1. Cut the onions in 2 lengthwise, then cut into thin slices.
2. In a casserole, brown the chicken pieces in olive oil. Remove the chicken and set aside.
3. In the same casserole sauté the ginger and onions until the onions become translucent. Return the browned chicken to the pot and add the salt and pepper. In a separate pan heat the liquid, add the saffron strands and then pour this over the chicken.
4. Simmer the chicken for 1 hour, then add the preserved lemon peel cut into thick strips. Let the dish cook for another 15 minutes.
5. Just before serving, chop the coriander (cilantro) and sprinkle over the chicken.

# Chicken with Tarragon

In France, chicken cooked with tarragon, or *Poulet à l'Estragon,* is a culinary tradition. This recipe is also delicious with guinea fowl.

O   suitable                          B   not suitable

A   omit the pepper                   AB   not suitable

SERVES 4

| | |
|---|---|
| 3½–4lb/1.6–1.8kg free-range chicken | Sea salt and freshly ground black pepper |
| 1 bunch tarragon | 1 fresh goat's cheese approx. ½lb/225g |
| 4 tbsp olive oil | 4 shallots, roughly chopped |

1.  Preheat the oven to 200°C/400°F/Gas mark 6.
2.  Separate the skin from the flesh under the breasts, drumsticks and legs as described in the Chicken with Lemon, Sage and Garlic recipe on page 126.
3.  Chop up all the tarragon leaves. Mix a third of the tarragon with 2 tablespoons of the olive oil. Using a teaspoon or your hands carefully push the mixture under the skin without tearing it.
4.  Season inside the cavity with salt and pepper.
5.  Mix the fresh goat's cheese with the shallots, the remaining tarragon, some salt and 2 tablespoons of olive oil, and stuff the bird. Sew up the cavity or use wooden skewers to keep the cavity closed.
6.  Rub the fowl with a little olive oil, place it breast side down in an ovenware dish and roast for 30 minutes. Half an hour later turn it over and cook for the last 30 minutes on its back.
7.  After 1 hour test the drumstick with the point of a sharp knife. If the juice is pink, it is not cooked. If the juice is transparent, the chicken is done. Take the dish out of the oven, cover the chicken and let it rest for 10 minutes to let the juices settle, then carve.
8.  Serve the chicken with its stuffing, and its juices.

## Ingredient Info: Tarragon

Read about tarragon in the section on herbs (page 64).

French tarragon is a most outstanding herb. Try it – fresh, of course – to believe it. In France it is used for fowl, eggs, sauces, salads, and to flavour vinegars and mustards. Tarragon has in the past been used to treat heart and liver problems, tumours and swellings. It is an excellent digestive aid that counteracts flatulence, poor appetite, parasites, weak and slow digestion. It is also well known as an anti-spasmodic and more specifically it works to stop hiccups.

# Chicken with Lemon, Sage and Garlic

**What makes this recipe special is that you put the flavouring under the chicken skin. It may sound complicated but it is actually very easy.**

| | | | |
|---|---|---|---|
| O | suitable | B | not suitable |
| A | omit the pepper | AB | not suitable |

SERVES 4

3½–4lb/1.6–1.8kg free-range chicken
1 lemon
3 tbsp olive oil
1 tsp dried thyme

20 fresh sage leaves
1 garlic clove
1 tsp honey
Sea salt and freshly ground black pepper

1. Juice half the lemon, add it to the olive oil, half the thyme, and 10 chopped sage leaves. This mixture is to go under the skin of the breasts, legs and drum sticks. Here is how to do it.
2. With the chicken lying on its back and the stomach cavity facing you, slip your fingers under the skin and gently make your way over the breasts, separating the skin from the meat. Now go along the drumsticks and legs, without tearing the skin. Place most of the mixture of olive and sage leaves in the gap between the meat and the skin. Add the honey to the leftover mixture, and coat the chicken skin with this.
3. Place half the lemon, the remaining sage leaves and thyme, and a pinch of salt in the stomach cavity.
4. Put the chicken breast-side down in an ovenware dish and place in a cold oven. Set the oven at 220°C/425°F/Gas mark 7. For the chicken to be golden all over, turn it over half way through the cooking. Baste the bird several times.
5. After 1 hour and 15 minutes test the drumstick with the point of a sharp knife. If the juice is pink, it is not cooked. If the juice is transparent, the chicken is done.
6. Before carving let the bird rest for 10 minutes for the juices to settle in the meat.

## Ingredient Info: Sage

Read about the benefits of sage in the section on herbs on page 63.

# Guinea Fowl with Sage

O    suitable

A    suitable

B    not suitable

AB   not suitable

SERVES 4

3lb/1.3kg guinea fowl with its liver

8 garlic cloves, crushed

1 tbsp dried thyme

6 fresh sage branches

Olive oil

Sea salt

STOCK:

Gizzard and neck from the fowl

2 garlic cloves, unpeeled

2 shallots, finely chopped

Sea salt

1 tbsp dried thyme

1½ cups/340ml water

3–4 leaves fresh sage

1. Preheat the oven to 200°C/400°F/Gas mark 6.
2. In a bowl mix the garlic, thyme, fincly chopped leaves from 3 sage branches, 2 tablespoons olive oil, and salt until you have a thick paste.
3. Separate the skin of the bird from the flesh (as described in the Chicken with Lemon, Sage and Garlic recipe opposite).
4. Using a teaspoon or your hands carefully place the garlic mixture, without tearing the skin, under the breasts, drumsticks and thighs.
5. Lightly salt the stomach cavity and place the remaining 3 sage branches and the liver in the cavity. Sew up the cavity.
6. Rub olive oil into the fowl and place breast-side down in an ovenware dish that has been coated with a little olive oil.
7. Place the bird in the oven. After 30 minutes turn the bird over onto its back and cook for another 30 minutes. When done, remove the bird from the oven and leave it to rest for 10 minutes to allow the juices to settle.
8. While the bird is cooking place the gizzard, neck, garlic cloves, shallots, salt and thyme in the water and simmer for 30 minutes. Add the sage leaves 3 minutes before the end. Allow it to steep for 10 minutes then pass the stock through a sieve. Return the stock to the pan and slowly reduce it to about ¾ cup/200ml.
9. Carve the fowl, reserving the juices. Add any juices to the stock and serve.

# Roast Venison

**For this recipe try to buy a roast that is long – similar to the French *filet de boeuf* – rather than a big chunk of meat.**

| O | suitable | B | suitable |
|---|----------|---|----------|
| A | not suitable | AB | not suitable |

SERVES 4

| | |
|---|---|
| 1¾lb/780g venison roast | Olive oil |
| 8 big shallots | Thyme, rosemary and oregano |

1. Preheat the oven to 220°C/425°F/Gas mark 7.
2. Cut the shallots into ¼ inch/5mm slices. Sauté the shallots until softened in the olive oil.
3. Choose an ovenware dish which is slightly longer than the roast. Scatter the shallots over the bottom of the dish, then add the meat and sprinkle the herbs over the meat. Roast in the oven for 15 minutes, then turn the meat over, lower the oven temperature to 190°C/375°F/Gas mark 5 and cook for another 15–30 minutes, according to whether you like medium rare, medium or well cooked meat.
4. Before cutting the meat, cover it and let it rest at room temperature for 10–15 minutes. This allows the juices to settle back into the meat.

# Marinated Roast Venison

**Marinating game will tenderize it and introduce subtle flavours into the meat.**

O   suitable

A   not suitable

B   suitable

AB   not suitable

SERVES 4

---

1¾lb/780g venison roast

Olive oil

MARINADE:

3 cups/750ml red wine

1 carrot, sliced

1 onion, finely sliced

5 garlic cloves, unpeeled

1 sprig fresh thyme

1 sprig fresh rosemary

1 bay leaf

10 juniper berries

Zest of ½ orange

3 tbsp olive oil

FOR THE ROUX:

1 tbsp clarified butter

1 tbsp spelt flour

1. Bring the wine to the boil. Add all the marinade ingredients, with the exception of the olive oil, and cook at low temperature for 30 minutes. Allow to cool, add the olive oil and mix well.
2. Place the venison in an earthenware dish, pour the marinade over the meat and cover. Rotate the meat twice a day for 1–2 days.
3. Remove the meat from the marinade and reserve the liquid. Dry the meat and set aside in a cool place for 24 hours.
4. In a cast iron or heavy casserole, brown the meat on all sides in the olive oil. Cover and cook slowly on low heat for 20–30 minutes (depending on the cut of the meat). Turn the meat over while cooking. Turn off the heat and leave covered for 15 minutes for the juices to settle.
5. Pour the marinade through a sieve, place the liquid in a saucepan and reduce it over medium to high heat.
6. Now prepare the sauce. Melt the clarified butter in a saucepan, add the flour and keep stirring with a wooden spoon until the mixture turns a rich brown colour. Add the marinade liquid, stirring constantly, and then the juices from the casserole. Add sea salt and freshly ground black pepper to taste.
7. Carve the meat and serve it with the rich dark sauce.

# Ostrich Steaks with Shallots and Red Wine

O  suitable

A  omit the pepper

B  suitable

AB  omit the pepper

SERVES 4

---

4 ostrich steaks, approximately 5oz/150g each

2 tbsp olive oil

8 medium shallots, finely chopped

4 tbsp red wine

Sea salt and freshly ground black pepper

1. Place the olive oil in a frying pan (skillet), add the shallots and cook until they become translucent. Remove the shallots and set aside.
2. Increase the heat, add the steaks and brown them on either side for 2–6 minutes depending how you like your meat. Place on serving plate.
3. Return the shallots to the pan, add the red wine, salt and pepper. Stir over the heat for 30 seconds, then pour over the meat. Serve immediately.

# Rabbit with Preserved Lemons

O  suitable

A  not suitable

B  suitable

AB  omit the pepper

SERVES 4

---

1 rabbit, cut into pieces

2 tbsp olive oil

2 garlic heads, cloves separated and peeled

2 tsp oregano

Sea salt and freshly ground black pepper

1 cup/250ml water or Chicken Stock (see recipe page 184)

1 Preserved Lemon (see recipe page 191)

½ bunch flat-leaf parsley, finely chopped

1. Place the olive oil in a large saucepan, add the rabbit pieces and cook until browned.
2. Add the garlic cloves, oregano, salt and pepper. Add the water or chicken stock and let the rabbit cook for 45 minutes.
3. Cut the preserved lemon into thin segments and add to the rabbit.
4. Continue cooking for 15 minutes. Serve sprinkled with the chopped parsley.

# Rabbit with Provençale Herbs

O  suitable

A  not suitable

B  suitable

AB  omit the pepper

SERVES 4

---

1 x 2½lb/1.1kg rabbit, cut into pieces

3 tbsp olive oil

2 garlic bulbs, cloves peeled

Sea salt and freshly ground black pepper

2 tbsp mustard, preferably with mustard seeds

HERBAL INFUSION:

4 cups/1 litre water

1 tbsp savory

1 tbsp thyme

1 tbsp rosemary

1. Boil the water with the 3 herbs and leave to steep for 10 minutes. Pour the liquid through a sieve and set aside.
2. In a cast iron or heavy pan slowly brown the rabbit pieces in the olive oil. The cooking must be slow so as not to dry the meat.
3. Remove the pieces from the pan and discard the excess fat.
4. Return the browned rabbit pieces to the pan, add garlic cloves, salt and pepper and half the herbal infusion.
5. Let the meat slowly simmer for 40 minutes. Keep checking that there is enough liquid and add more if necessary.
6. Remove the rabbit pieces and set aside. With a hand-held blender, blend the garlic in the leftover liquid. This will produce a rich and thick sauce.
7. Add the mustard to the sauce, then the rabbit pieces and gently reheat before serving.

# Wild Duck

**There is no simpler way of preparing wild duck. The taste of the animal is so superb that it is sufficient on its own.**

O   suitable

A   not suitable

B   not suitable

AB  not suitable

SERVES 4

2 wild ducks, 1½lb/675 g each

Olive oil

Sea salt and freshly ground pepper

1. Preheat the oven to 220°C/425°F/Gas mark 7.
2. Rub the duck skin with a small amount of olive oil. Sprinkle salt and pepper on the inside and outside of the ducks.
3. Place in an ovenware dish just large enough to take the ducks.
4. Lay them in the dish breast-side down and place in the oven.
5. After 15 minutes turn them over and cook for another 15 minutes.
6. Remove the ducks from the oven and wait 10 minutes for the juices to settle before serving. Serve on hot plates.

# tofu and tempeh

Tofu is a bean curd made from soaked soya beans that are blended with hot water, then drained to extract the soya milk. The milk is cooked for 7 minutes and then a coagulant is added to curdle it. The taste of tofu is bland but it takes up any flavours with which it comes in contact. It does not require any further cooking so you can use it raw or, of course, you may also cook it.

Tofu is an excellent source of protein for type As and to a slightly lesser degree for type AB. Os may eat some tofu but should get most of their protein from red meat. Bs should avoid tofu.

Another very healthy way of eating soya beans is by consuming fermented soya bean products. As well as tempeh, try miso, tamari, shoyu, natto and okara (unfortunately the latter two are not as widely available as the rest). Fermenting foods greatly enhances their enzyme content. Enzymes are needed for every chemical reaction in the body and by including these cultured soya products in your diet you will increase your enzyme intake and thereby improve your health. Tamari, according to research published in April 1992 in the journal *Cancer Research*, was shown to inhibit the development of cancer in laboratory animals. Miso is also reputed to have anti-cancer effects, antioxidant activity and to lower cholesterol.

Tempeh was originally developed on the Indonesian island of Java. Soya beans are cooked and then inoculated with a mould that goes to work on the beans at a certain temperature for 30 hours. This produces enzymes that give the beans their distinctive flavour and decrease the antinutrient factors in soya.

Tempeh is a good source of protein for As and ABs, and provides antioxidants and fibre. Although tempeh is known to be rich in vitamin $B_{12}$, it cannot be relied upon to improve one's vitamin $B_{12}$ status. This is because the amount of vitamin $B_{12}$ varies greatly with each batch and it is also not yet known whether $B_{12}$ from tempeh is well absorbed by the body. If you are a vegetarian and in need of vitamin $B_{12}$ use a supplement.

# Marinated Tofu Brochettes with Thyme and Oregano

**This refined way of serving tofu is perfect for a light vegetable protein meal.**

O   suitable

A   omit the tomatoes and (bell) peppers

B   not suitable

AB   omit the (bell) peppers

SERVES 4

1lb/450g firm tofu

8 cherry tomatoes

2 green or red (bell) peppers, cut into
   1 inch/2.5cm pieces

2 medium courgettes (zucchini), cut into
   1 inch/2.5cm chunks

4 green onions, cut lengthwise into 1 inch/2.5cm
   pieces

1 fennel bulb, cut into 1 inch/2.5cm pieces

BROCHETTE MARINADE:

4 tbsp olive oil

2 tbsp freshly squeezed lemon juice

2 garlic cloves, crushed

½ tbsp dried thyme

½ tbsp dried oregano

1 bay leaf

1 tsp sea salt

1.  Mix all the ingredients for the marinade together and set aside.
2.  Cut the tofu into 1 inch/2.5cm squares and marinate in the prepared mixture for several hours – 24 hours if possible – in the refrigerator. Turn the pieces over in the marinade occasionally.
3.  Assemble the brochettes on 8–10 inch/20–25cm long wooden skewers (2 per person), alternating the vegetables and tofu to give a colourful result. Place the brochettes on greaseproof (waxed) paper on a baking sheet. Brush all over the brochettes with the marinade and grill (broil) until all sides of the tofu are golden, 10–15 minutes.
4.  Serve hot accompanied with a mixed green salad or with brown rice and some of the marinade. Use any leftover marinade for steamed vegetables, rice or even as a salad dressing.

# Marinated Tempeh

O   suitable           B   not suitable

A   suitable           AB  suitable

SERVES 4

¾lb/340g tempeh in cake or sausage form

MARINADE:

2 tbsp tamari

3 tbsp lemon juice

1 large garlic clove, finely chopped

Fresh ginger root, the size of a nutmeg, cut into fine matchsticks

1. Steam the tempeh for 15 minutes.
2. During this time mix the ingredients for the marinade.
3. Cut the tempeh into ½ inch/1cm slices, then cut each slice into four pieces.
4. Place the tempeh in the marinade and let it absorb all the flavours for at least 30 minutes.
5. Serve warm or at room temperature with Basil Sauce or Fresh Coriander Sauce (see pages 143 and 139).

# Marinated Tofu

O   suitable           B   not suitable

A   suitable           AB  suitable

SERVES 4

¾lb/340g tofu

MARINADE:

2 tbsp tamari

2 tbsp lemon juice

1 large garlic clove, finely chopped

Fresh ginger root, the size of a nutmeg, cut into fine matchsticks

1. Mix the ingredients for the marinade together.
2. Cut the tofu in ¾ inch/2cm cubes. Add to the marinade and let the flavours seep through the tofu for at least an hour.

# Pan-Fried Tempeh

**Here are some crispy protein "fries". This is the easiest way to prepare tempeh. It always needs to be cooked – either steamed, simmered in stock or pan-fried.**

O   suitable                     B   not suitable
A   suitable                     AB  suitable

SERVES 4

½lb/225g tempeh                  Sea salt
2 tbsp olive oil

1.  Heat the olive oil in a pan. Add the tempeh and fry on each side for 5 minutes until golden brown.
2.  Remove from pan and drain on kitchen paper. Sprinkle with sea salt and serve hot.

# sauces

The sauces and dressings featured in this section are virtually all made with raw ingredients. They make use of the goodness of olive oil and walnut oil, of fresh herbs and raw garlic. Fresh sauces made in this way contribute to your health by providing valuable nutrients, phytochemicals and enzymes. They also add zest to satisfy our taste buds. As an added bonus, the culinary herbs used in some of the sauces help with digestion. As you will have discovered in the earlier section on culinary herbs, they have some amazing health benefits. One Japanese researcher has discovered, for instance, that coriander (cilantro) eaten in large quantities has the ability to remove toxic metals such as mercury from the central nervous system – a difficult area of the body to detoxify.

Make your sauces and dressings just before eating. Fresh is the key word when eating for health.

# Aïoli

**This is a quick way to make a garlic mayonnaise. If you follow the instructions exactly, you will have a successful aïoli in a few seconds. You will need an electric hand-held blender and a jar or glass the width of the base of the blender.**

| O | suitable | B | suitable |
|---|---|---|---|
| A | omit the pepper and use vinegar-free mustard and lemon juice | AB | omit the pepper and use vinegar-free mustard and lemon juice |

3 garlic cloves, roughly chopped
1 organic egg, extra fresh
1 tsp Dijon-style mustard
1 pinch sea salt
1 twist of the pepper grinder
1 tsp wine vinegar, cider vinegar or lemon juice
1 cup/250ml extra virgin olive oil

EXTRA SEASONING:
1 tsp vinegar or more according to taste
Sea salt and freshly ground black pepper

*All the ingredients must be at room temperature*

1.  Place the 7 ingredients in the jar or glass in the order given – garlic, egg, mustard, salt, pepper, vinegar or lemon juice and oil. Don't stir.
2.  Slowly introduce the blade of the hand-held blender to the bottom of the jar. Switch it on and with a spiral movement upwards bring the blade to the top until all the oil is incorporated. The aïoli is done.
3.  Add extra seasoning if necessary. You can keep the aïoli several days in the refrigerator. Don't stir it when it is cold as the emulsion will break down. Allow it to reach room temperature, then stir if necessary.

## Ingredient Info: Garlic

Garlic is one of the wonder foods of the world. Its general antimicrobial activity fights all sorts of organisms: bacteria, virus, fungus and parasites. However, you must eat it raw to benefit from this effect.

Garlic is also a boon for cardiovascular health – it lowers blood pressure, reduces cholesterol and prevents clotting. Eating five fresh garlic cloves a day can dramatically lower your blood cholesterol and by eating two cloves a day you can maintain a good acceptable level. Both raw and cooked garlic work for a healthy heart. To maintain health, eat garlic regularly in your raw and cooked dishes. Chewing fresh parsley will neutralize garlic breath.

# Fresh Coriander Sauce

For this recipe you will need a hand-held blender that has its own glass container or alternatively use a jar or glass as wide as the base of the blender. This sauce can accompany many dishes such as Braised Beef, Fish Terrine, tempeh and steamed fish and vegetables.

O   suitable

A   suitable

B   use walnuts

AB  use walnuts or pine nuts

SERVES 4

---

I big handful/50g fresh coriander (cilantro) leaves

2 garlic cloves, roughly chopped

2 tbsp roasted pine nuts or walnuts, or tahini

4 tbsp extra virgin olive oil

I pinch fine sea salt

1. Wash and dry the coriander (cilantro) leaves.
2. Put all the ingredients in the jar, with the exception of the coriander (cilantro). Mix using the hand-held blender until you have a pesto-like paste.
3. Add the coriander (cilantro) and mix until the herb is well incorporated.
4. Adjust the seasoning if necessary.

## Ingredient Info: Coriander (cilantro)

Read about coriander (cilantro) in the section on herbs on page 62.

# Ginger and Tamari Sauce

**This sauce is excellent with grilled (broiled) tuna or cold chicken and turkey. You can use chopsticks and dip each mouthful in the sauce.**

| | | | |
|---|---|---|---|
| O | suitable | B | suitable |
| A | suitable | AB | suitable |

SERVES 4

---

½ cup/125ml tamari

1 garlic clove, crushed

1 piece of fresh ginger root the size of a nutmeg, finely chopped

1 tsp dry sherry or Noilly Prat, optional

2 green onions with their greenery

1. Pour the tamari into a bowl.
2. Add the crushed garlic, the finely chopped ginger and the sherry or Noilly Prat. You can prepare the sauce in advance up to this point.
3. Cut the green onions into very fine slices at a slant. Just before serving add to the sauce and pour into 4 individual dipping bowls.

## Ingredient Info: Ginger

Read about ginger in the Green Tea with Ginger recipe on page 161.

# Parsley Sauce

Parsley has excellent antioxidant properties and a soothing effect on the digestive tract, so everyone should eat lots of it. This recipe is an excellent way of doing just that. The sauce is delicious on rye or spelt toast or as an accompaniment to fish or cold chicken. For this recipe you will need an electric hand-held blender and a jar or glass as wide as the base of the blender.

O   suitable                       B   suitable
A   suitable                       AB  suitable

SERVES 4

½ cup/125ml extra virgin olive oil          I tsp sea salt
2 garlic cloves, finely chopped             2 cups/500ml flat-leaf parsley without stems

1.   Pour the olive oil into the jar or glass, add the garlic and salt, and blend. Slowly add the parsley leaves, a small handful at a time, until the leaves are all incorporated. Check the seasoning.

## Ingredient Info: Parsley

Read about parsley in the section on herbs on page 62.

# Soya Yogurt Dill Sauce

**This sauce is a good accompaniment for fish dishes.**

O  suitable

A  omit the pepper

B  not suitable

AB  omit the pepper

SERVES 4

---

1 cup/250ml unsweetened soya yogurt

1 tbsp extra virgin olive oil

½ bunch dill, very finely chopped

Zest and juice of ½ non-treated lime

Sea salt and freshly ground black pepper

1.  Mix all the ingredients together and serve.

## Ingredient Info: Dill

Read about dill on page 62.

# Summer Salad Dressing

**This light dressing is perfect for tender summer salad leaves. For extra taste we add flat-leaf parsley, chopped chives, fresh coriander (cilantro) leaves, piquant-tasting nasturtium leaves and flowers, tarragon, purple basil – whatever is available. The fresh summer herbs at the markets inspire us.**

O  use lemon juice

A  use lemon juice and omit the pepper

B  suitable

AB  use lemon juice and omit the pepper

SERVES 4

---

Summer herbs

3 tbsp extra virgin olive oil

1 tbsp balsamic vinegar, red wine vinegar or
    lemon juice

1 tsp vinegar-free mustard

Fine sea salt and freshly ground black pepper

1.  Mix all the ingredients together and serve on the summer greens.

# Sweet Basil Sauce

**Green sauces that include a large amount of herbs are a delicious means of obtaining the health benefits of herbs. This sauce can accompany many dishes such as Braised Beef, Fish Mousse, tempeh and steamed vegetables. For this recipe you will need an electric hand-held blender and a jar or glass as wide as the base of the blender.**

| | | | |
|---|---|---|---|
| O | suitable | B | use walnuts |
| A | suitable | AB | use walnuts or pine nuts |

SERVES 4

---

1 big handful/50g sweet basil leaves
2 garlic cloves, roughly chopped
2 tbsp toasted pine nuts or walnuts, or tahini

4 tbsp extra virgin olive oil
1 pinch fine sea salt

1. Wash and dry the basil leaves.
2. Put all the ingredients in the jar, with the exception of the basil. Mix using the hand-held blender until you have a pesto-like paste.
3. Add the basil and mix until well incorporated.
4. Check the seasoning.

## Nutritional Info: Basil

Read about basil on page 63.

# Vinaigrette Dressing

**This is one of our favourite salad dressings. Occasionally we vary the oils by using fresh walnut oil, grilled walnut oil, hazelnut oil and so on. We have noticed how most of our friends allow themselves an extra piece of bread to clean up their salad dressing – a success indeed!**

O   use the lemon juice

A   omit the pepper and use lemon juice

B   omit the sesame oil, although a few drops will not harm and add such a delightful flavour

AB   omit the pepper and use lemon juice. Leave out the sesame oil, although a few drops will not harm and add such a delightful flavour

SERVES 4

---

1 tsp vinegar-free mustard
3 tbsp extra virgin olive oil
1 tbsp balsamic vinegar or lemon juice
1 garlic clove, crushed

A few drops toasted sesame oil
A few drops tamari or soya sauce
Fine sea salt and freshly ground black pepper

1. Put the mustard, oil, vinegar or lemon juice in the bottom of the salad bowl. Stir until it thickens, then add the remaining ingredients. Check the seasoning.
2. If you put the serving spoon and fork criss-cross in the bowl, you can then add the salad without it falling into the dressing. Just before eating the salad, toss the leaves in the dressing.

# desserts

Desserts are part of life rather than part of health. Unfortunately, for many people they have become part of everyday life and are sometimes eaten several times a day. This is largely because the more sugar you eat the more you want to eat. Sugar depletes the body of valuable nutrients needed for proper sugar metabolism and when these nutrients are lacking the body calls for more sugar.

Sugar-laden foods deliver calories to the system that are very quickly absorbed and they therefore almost immediately relieve the need for food. The feelings of hunger may be satisfied but because they lack fibre these foods do not make you feel full – this means it's easy to eat lots of them. This is especially true of children, who are often lazy when it comes to chewing.

Overconsumption of sugar has been linked with a weakened immune system, elevated blood fat levels, elevated uric acid levels leading to gout, behavioural and learning problems in adults and children, diabetes, obesity, hypertension, yeast overgrowth, impaired digestion etc.

If sugar is a craving for you, or if you think your health problems could be related to heavy sugar consumption, cut it out with the help of a health care professional. He or she can give you specialized advice for your personal situation. Begin by reducing the amount of sugar in your diet. Consider certain nutrients such as zinc, chromium, magnesium, biotin and vanadium to help you out. Zinc is an important one to consider as it is vital to have sensitive taste buds. If you lack zinc in your diet you may be adding more sugar (and salt) because your sense of taste is very weak. You may need to include more protein (meat, fish, poultry, egg, tofu) with each meal and even with each snack (try nuts, seeds and yogurt in accordance with your blood group). Reducing sugar may be difficult in the beginning but the minerals and the added protein should help reduce the cravings.

Our recipes include desserts made with as little sweetener as possible. We have used brown sugar, honey and maple syrup mainly because each imparts a different taste to food. However, there is really no such thing as a healthy sweetener. Sugar in all its forms should be kept within good limits. Molasses can be used by all blood types as a sweetener and it does contain a reasonably good amount of iron and calcium.

Remember your main foods should be meats, poultry, fish, vegetables, fruits, grains, seeds, beans, lentils, and milk products – all in accordance with your blood group. You will have much more energy if desserts are kept as a treat. Instilling the concept that sweet foods are a rare treat (and not part of the daily diet) is one of the best health habits you can pass on to your children.

# Apple, Walnut and Maple Syrup Pie

**This pie is a treat.**

O    not suitable            B    suitable
A    not suitable            AB   not suitable

SERVES 6

---

| |  |
|---|---|
| 1 thin pie crust (see basic recipe page 193) for a 10 inch/25cm pie dish | 1½ cups/200g freshly shelled chopped walnuts |
| 4 eating (dessert) apples, peeled, cored and cut into thin slices | 1 cup/250ml maple syrup |
| | ½ cup/125ml double (heavy) cream |

1. Preheat the oven to 190°C/375° F/Gas mark 5.
2. Toast the walnuts in the oven, turning them every now and then, until they become golden and fragrant. This will take about 8–10 minutes.
3. Arrange the apple slices in the pastry shell. Start on the outside and work inward, overlapping the slices.
4. Bake the pie for 35–40 minutes until golden.
5. While the pie is in the oven, reduce the maple syrup by half over low heat. Add the cream and cook for 10 minutes, stirring constantly.
6. Remove the mixture from the heat, add the walnuts and stir until the mixture cools down. Pour over the pie and serve at room temperature.

## Ingredient Info: Walnuts

The walnut is a very healthy nut. It is one of the rare ones to contain the valuable linolenic acid, also called omega-3 oil. Our western diets are lacking in this family of oils and a variety of health problems are linked with this deficiency. Another top source of linolenic acid is linseed oil. Although walnuts are high in fats, they contain beneficial fats. They are also a good source of minerals and fibre.

As walnuts are high in linolenic acid they become rancid very easily and should be bought in their shells and cracked just before eating. They are also a good source of protein and minerals. Walnuts can be eaten by all blood types.

# Autumn Apple Pie

O  suitable

A  suitable

B  not suitable

AB  not suitable

SERVES 4—6

1 pie crust shell (see basic recipe page 193) for a
    10 inch/25cm pie dish
5–6 cooking apples (about 800g), peeled, cored
    and cut into thin slices
2 tbsp clarified butter (see recipe page 187)
1 tbsp brown sugar

TOPPING:
¾ cup/100g hazelnuts, chopped
1 tbsp clarified butter
1 tbsp brown sugar

1.  Preheat the oven to 190° C/375°F/Gas mark 5.
2.  Arrange the apple slices in circles on the pastry shell.
3.  Sprinkle small pieces of clarified butter and sugar over the apples. Bake for 25 minutes.
4.  Distribute the hazelnuts, the clarified butter (in small pieces) and the brown sugar over the apples. Bake for another 10 minutes, ensuring that the hazelnuts do not burn.
5.  Serve at room temperature.

## Ingredient Info: Apples

An apple a day keeps the doctor away as the saying goes. But why? Apples are the friend of your cardiovascular system. Eating 2 raw apples a day has been shown to lower LDL cholesterol (the bad one) and raise HDL cholesterol (the good one). And thanks to their diuretic effect apples can help lower blood pressure.

If you are constipated eat at least 2 apples a day. If you have diarrhoea cook your apples. Well chewed, raw apple has a beneficial effect on stomach disorders, digestive problems, slow digestion and even dysentery.

The pectin in apples is perhaps their most valuable component. Pectin is an excellent detoxifying agent, assisting the body in the elimination of all sorts of toxins. It also encourages the bowel muscles to keep moving.

An apple fast for one or two days every now and then is a good way to help your body in its detoxification process. You will get the most benefit from eating your apples raw or juicing them. But you will also reap some benefit from baked apples.

# Chocolate Delight

**A quick and easy chocolate dessert. It can be decorated with grated orange zest, chopped candied orange peel or candied ginger. For a bit of added flavour mix in 2 tablespoons of instant coffee to make a mocha dessert.**

O   suitable

A   suitable

B   not suitable

AB  suitable

SERVES 6

---

1¼ cups/300ml unsweetened soya milk

1 vanilla bean

9oz/250g 70% cocoa bittersweet/dark chocolate

3 organic eggs

1 tbsp Grand Marnier liqueur

1.  In a small saucepan slowly heat the milk with the vanilla bean until boiling. Allow to steep for 10 minutes then remove the vanilla bean.
2.  Break the chocolate into pieces and place it in the hot milk to melt.
3.  Mix the eggs, one by one, and the Grand Marnier into the milk until the mixture is well blended.
4.  Pour the mixture into 6 little ramekins and refrigerate for at least 3 hours.

# Dark Plum Pie

| O | suitable | B | suitable |
|---|----------|---|----------|
| A | use clarified butter | AB | use clarified butter |

SERVES 4—6

---

1 thin pie crust (see basic recipe page 193) for a
    10 inch/25cm pie dish
2lb/1kg dark red oval plums
½ tsp ground ginger

6 green cardamom pods
2 tbsp/25g butter or clarified butter, cut into
    pieces (see recipe page 187)
2 tbsp brown sugar

1.  Preheat the oven to 190°C/375° F/Gas mark 5.
2.  Remove the cardamom seeds from the pods. Pound the seeds in a mortar and heat them slightly under the grill (broiler) to enhance the aroma.
3.  Cut the plums in 2 lengthwise and discard the stones. Arrange the cut plums skin side down on the pie crust, working from the outside into the centre.
4.  Sprinkle the ground cardamom and sugar on the fruit. Scatter pieces of butter on the plums.
5.  Bake the pie for 30–35 minutes until the pastry is golden. The fruit will become a dark red. Serve at room temperature.

## Ingredient Info: Cardamom

Cardamom is an exquisite spice commonly used in Indian cooking and in the Ayurvedic healing system. Its taste is pungent, slightly acidic and warm. The latter characteristic makes it warming to the body. The tiny cardamom seeds come in a pod. Look for the green ones, they are the best. Cardamom can be used both with and without the pod. However, always buy it in pods, as it loses its aroma and its quality very quickly if already ground.

Cardamom seeds can be chewed after a meal to refresh the breath and whiten the teeth, so it's useful for those who eat lots of garlic. Cardamom is effective for relieving flatulence, and strengthens the digestive system. It soothes stomach aches, intestinal spasms and colic, and is also used for ailments of the genito-urinary tract such as cystitis and urinary incontinence. This wonderful-tasting spice can also lift your spirits if you are feeling depressed.

To combat wind and bloating, make an infusion of cardamom. Crush the seeds of 2–3 cardamom pods in a mortar, add to a cup of boiling water and infuse for 10 minutes. Add a bit of honey if desired. Drink several times a day.

# Pear Fruit Salad

**Adding ginger imparts pungency to the delicate, sweet taste of pears.**

O  suitable

A  suitable

B  suitable

AB suitable

SERVES 6

---

6 ripe pears

Juice and zest of 1 non-treated lemon

2 tbsp brown sugar

½ tsp ground ginger

3 tbsp water

1. Peel the pears, cut them into quarters and remove the cores. Cut each quarter into three pieces lengthwise and place in a salad bowl. Drizzle some of the lemon juice over the pears so they don't become brown.
2. Mix the remaining lemon juice with the zest, sugar, ginger and water. Pour over the pears and mix very carefully with your hands so as not to damage the pears. Serve at room temperature.

# Plum Crumble

**This crumble may of course be used with numerous other fruit such as apples, cherries, apricots, berries etc.**

O   suitable

A   use clarified butter

B   suitable

AB   use clarified butter

SERVES 4

2lbs/1kg little summer plums (Mirabelle), cut in 2

Juice of ½ a lemon

1 tsp ground ginger

1 tbsp arrowroot – add brown sugar if the fruit is
    tart

¾ cup/100g spelt flour

5 tbsp rolled oats, optional

1 cup/100g ground almonds

½ cup/50 g brown sugar

½ cup/125g butter or clarified butter, cut into
    small cubes (see recipe page 187)

Zest of 1 lemon

1.   Preheat the oven to 190°C/375° F/Gas mark 5.
2.   Butter an ovenware dish and put in the plums.
3.   Mix the lemon juice, ginger and arrowroot and pour over the fruit.
4.   Place the flour, oats, ground almonds, sugar, butter and lemon zest in a bowl and mix with your fingertips. The mixture must remain light.
5.   Spread the topping over the fruit and bake for 35 minutes until golden.

# Poached Pears in Citrus Juice and Grand Marnier

O   use grapefruit juice

A   use grapefruit juice

B   use either orange or grapefruit juice

AB  use grapefruit juice

SERVES 6

---

6 firm whole ripe pears, peeled and stems left on

2 cups/500ml freshly squeezed orange or
    grapefruit juice

Juice of 1 lime

Zest of 1 orange, cut into fine strips

3 tbsp Grand Marnier or Cointreau liqueur

1 tbsp honey

1. Soak the strips of orange zest in boiling water for 3 minutes, drain and set aside.
2. Place the pears, standing upright, in a large saucepan. Pour the orange and lime juice over the fruit. Add the orange zest, cover and simmer until pears are tender – about 15 minutes. Check they are cooked with the sharp point of a knife.
3. Remove the pears and place in a serving dish.
4. Add the honey to the juice and reduce the liquid over medium heat for 15 minutes. Heat the Grand Marnier or Cointreau. Once boiling, flambé the liquid. This eliminates the alcohol. Add this to the juice and pour over the pears. Serve at room temperature.

## Ingredient Info: Orange and Grapefruit

These citrus fruits, native to south Asia, have been shown to lower cholesterol levels. In order to achieve this you must eat the pulp, the membranes and possibly the white pith. The pectin seems to be the active compound, working in synergy with other components in the fruit. So if you squeeze your own orange or grapefruit juice make sure you also eat the bits that you might normally throw away. Grapefruits seem to be the more effective of the two.

# Quick Mango Sherbet

This sherbet is prepared in the reverse order to a traditional sherbet. Instead of freezing the fruit mixture, you use frozen fruit. The advantage of this is that it only takes a few minutes to prepare. If you can't find frozen mangoes in your supermarket buy fresh ones, cut them in half, remove the stone and freeze for several hours. This is a delicious dessert that's always greatly appreciated by guests.

| | | | |
|---|---|---|---|
| O | omit the cream | B | suitable |
| A | not suitable | AB | not suitable |

SERVES 4

---

1lb/450g frozen mango pieces
½ banana
Juice of half a lemon

2 tbsp brown sugar, optional
1 tbsp double (heavy) cream, optional

1. Take the frozen mango pieces out of the freezer approximately 10 minutes before making the sherbet.
2. Blend the mango pieces in the food processor. Add banana, lemon juice, sugar and cream.
3. Spoon into individual bowls and serve immediately as the sherbet will melt quite quickly.

# Raspberry Sherbet

In traditional sherbets, the fruit mixture is frozen; here we use frozen fruit to speed up the recipe. If you prefer not to use ready-frozen raspberries, buy fresh ones and freeze them for several hours.

| | | | |
|---|---|---|---|
| O | suitable | B | suitable |
| A | suitable | AB | suitable |

SERVES 4

1 lb/450g frozen raspberries
4 tbsp brown sugar

5 tbsp lemon juice

1. Ten minutes before making the sherbet take the raspberries out of the freezer – 15 minutes if they are whole and not broken into pieces.
2. Pulse all the ingredients in a food processor. Scrape down the sides of the food processor bowl and pulse again to obtain a thick mass of sherbet. If the raspberries are small and not very sweet, you might need to add a little more sugar. The less sugar the better.
3. Serve immediately.

# Sourdough Buckwheat or Spelt Pancakes

**These slightly raised pancakes can be served as a filling dessert or for a Sunday breakfast. They are also good served as a light meal with a savoury accompaniment such as goat's cheese and a mixed green salad.**

| | | | |
|---|---|---|---|
| O | use soya milk | B | use spelt flour |
| A | suitable | AB | use spelt flour |

MAKES 30 SMALL PANCAKES

2 cups/500ml soya or goat's milk

2 tbsp dried organic sourdough starter

1 tbsp sugar

2 cups/280g buckwheat or spelt flour

½ tsp salt

4 organic eggs

Clarified butter for the griddle
(see recipe page 187)

TO SERVE:
Maple syrup, honey, lemon juice, etc.

1. Heat the milk in a small saucepan until it reaches body temperature.
2. Using a whisk, mix a quarter of the milk, the dried sourdough starter and sugar. Let the starter stand for 10 minutes.
3. Add the leftover milk, flour, salt and the eggs, one by one. The consistency should be like liquid whipping cream. If it is too thick you can add more milk or even some water.
4. To allow the batter to rise, cover the mixture with a dish towel and set aside for a few hours in a warm place or overnight in the refrigerator. The dough should double in size.
5. To cook the pancakes, heat a large pancake griddle. To test if it's hot enough, sprinkle a few drops of water in the pan – if they bounce off it's ready. Grease with clarified butter.
6. Using a small ladle pour in enough batter to make as many 3 inch/7cm pancakes as possible. Cook the pancakes for 2–3 minutes until small bubbles appear on the surface, then flip them over and cook the other side for 1–2 minutes. The pancakes can be kept warm in the oven, but they are so much better eaten as soon as they are made.
7. Serve the pancakes with maple syrup, honey, fresh fruit purée, apple sauce or fresh fruit, according to your blood group.

# Spicy Peaches in Red Wine

**A delicious alternative to peaches and cream.**

O  suitable

A  suitable

B  suitable

AB  suitable

SERVES 4

6 peaches, yellow or white

½ tsp ground ginger

2 tbsp brown sugar

Grated zest of 1 non-treated lemon

1 cup/250ml light red wine

1.  Mix the ginger, sugar and lemon zest with the red wine.
2.  Remove the skin from the peaches. If they are ripe the peel should pull off easily. Cut them into slices and remove the stone.
3.  Add the peach slices to the red wine, and serve.

# Summer Red Fruit

**This dessert is a lovely alternative to red berries and cream.**

| O | suitable | B | suitable |
|---|----------|---|----------|
| A | suitable | AB | suitable |

SERVES 4

---

1lb/450g strawberries  
½ cup/150g raspberries  
½ cup/150g redcurrants  
Juice of ½ lime  

3 tbsp brown sugar  
1 tsp ground ginger  
¾ cup/2g agar agar  
1 tbsp arrowroot  

1. Place all the ingredients, with the exception of the raspberries, in a saucepan and bring to the boil, stirring constantly. Let the fruit simmer for 5 minutes.
2. Add the raspberries.
3. Pour the mixture into small serving bowls or ramekins, let them cool and then refrigerate.
4. Half an hour before serving, take the bowls out of the refrigerator.

## Ingredient info: Agar Agar and Arrowroot

Agar agar is a product derived from a red seaweed. It is native to the Pacific coasts of China, Japan and South Africa. It is commonly used as a thickening agent in food preparation and thickens more quickly than gelatine. It is useful for stimulating intestinal transit.

Arrowroot is a very fine textured powder used for thickening sauces. It comes from a rhizome native to northern South America and the Caribbean. Traditionally it was used by the Arawak of South America as an antidote to arrow poisons. In our civilization we use it to relieve acidity and digestive disorders.

# drinks

In this section we have included two warm drinks: Dandelion Coffee with Cardamom and Green Tea with Ginger. Dandelion coffee is an excellent substitute for coffee, while green tea is an excellent substitute for black tea. Coffee and black tea in excessive quantities (and for some people in small quantities), can have a detrimental influence on health. Both contain caffeine, which stimulates the adrenal glands thereby increasing blood sugar levels and providing a "lift". The nervous system is also stimulated. When caffeine intake becomes a habit and is repeated several times a day symptoms of toxicity can occur: insomnia, anxiety, nervousness, premenstrual syndrome, rapid heartbeat, heartburn, increased blood pressure etc ... If you are seriously hooked on caffeine you may need to seek the expertise of a nutritionist to help you break the habit.

The drinks we offer here as substitutes both have outstanding health properties (read about these in the information accompanying the recipes). The added benefit of replacing coffee with dandelion coffee is that it will help with the detoxification process. Although green tea does contain caffeine it has less than a third of the amount found in black tea and the general health benefits far outweigh the caffeine content (see page 161).

Also included in this section are four vegetable juices that suit all four blood types. However, each one is particularly good for one blood type. Juicing is one of the best ways to enjoy your fruit and veg, so experiment and use your imagination to concoct some of your own favourites.

# Dandelion Coffee with Cardamom

**Cardamom gives this drink a very pleasant aromatic taste. Roasted dandelion root is available in health food stores. You may also make this drink with instant organic dandelion coffee. Add the cardamom and leave it to sit for 10 minutes before drinking.**

| O | suitable | B | suitable |
|---|----------|---|----------|
| A | suitable | AB | suitable |

SERVES 2

6 cardamom pods
1 tbsp roasted dandelion root

2 cups/500ml fresh or filtered water

1. Squeeze one end of the cardamom pods to open them slightly (this allows more flavour to escape).
2. Place all the ingredients in a pan and bring to the boil. Turn off the heat and leave it to sit for 10 minutes. Serve as is or with milk (B, AB) or soya milk (O, A, AB).

## Ingredient Info: Cardamom

Read about cardamom in the Dark Plum Pie recipe on page 150.

# Green Tea with Ginger

**This drink puts two oriental health marvels together – ginger and green tea.**

O  suitable                                    B  suitable
A  suitable                                   AB  suitable

I SERVING

4 slices of fresh ginger root with skin          I cup fresh boiling water
½ tsp green tea

1.  Pour the boiling water over the ginger root and steep for 10 minutes. Add the
    green tea and allow it to steep for another 2 minutes. Strain and drink.

## Ingredient Info: Ginger

Ginger is used in many forms: fresh or green ginger, dried ginger, candied ginger,
ground ginger, preserved ginger. When you buy fresh ginger root, look for nice plump
rhizomes with a light coloured skin. In India, ginger is called the great medicine.

Traditionally ginger is used to strengthen weak digestion; stimulate the appetite;
relieve wind, nausea, vomiting and spasms; cure impotency; liven up a waning sex
life; cure the common cold, and as a pain reliever for headaches, joint pain and
toothache.

Human studies have shown it to act as an anti-inflammatory for arthritic conditions (good for Os) and headache and to be a very effective remedy against nausea
and motion sickness. Animal studies suggest it may be of use for lowering cholesterol (good for As and ABs), preventing ulcer formation (good for Os), relieving
pain and colic, and preventing blood clotting (good for As and ABs).

Ginger reduces gastric secretion in the stomach which is of benefit to Os, who
have a tendency towards too much acidity. Ginger also has antibacterial activity,
making it specially good for Bs, who are susceptible to bacterial infection.

As you can see ginger has something for every blood group, so make it a part of
your diet.

## Ingredient Info: Green tea

Despite there being hundreds of varieties of teas, all of them, no matter what their
colour, come from the same plant. The difference in colour is due to the method of
preparation: blue-green, red and black teas are fermented for a specific length of
time, while green tea is not fermented at all. The different varieties of green tea
depend on the area it originates from.

What interests us here are the health benefits of green tea, which has been shown in studies to have anti-cancer and cardiovascular effects. It contains polyphenols that have been shown to have greater antioxidant potential than vitamin C and E. The fermented teas, most of which are what we call black tea in the West, are oxidized. This destroys most of the beneficial activity of the polyphenols in tea. In addition, green tea could increase the antioxidant enzymes already present in the body. Green tea seems to give most protection against cancer of the digestive tract, the lungs and breast cancer. Green tea may also have cardiovascular effects by lowering cholesterol levels and high blood pressure.

You should drink at least 3 cups of green tea per day to benefit from its protective effects. If you shop around you will quickly notice a great variation in quality and price. One of the most highly respected Chinese tea masters, Yu Hui Tseng, recommends infusing most green teas for 2 minutes in water that has cooled down to 70°C (158°F). Another way to go about this, if you do not have the patience to wait, is to pour a little cold water on the tea before adding boiling water. This procedure prevents the leaves being scalded as green tea is quite fragile. If possible buy the best quality green teas as these use the bud and top leaves of the plant, the parts with the highest concentration of polyphenols.

Green tea is very good for all blood types but is especially useful for As and ABs, who have a higher risk of cancer and cardiovascular disease.

Green tea has also been shown to help in the fight against micro-organisms, making it particularly good for Bs. It strengthens the various cells of our immune system so they will be more effective in combating bacteria and viruses; and it has also been shown to "inhibit the growth and reproduction of many species of bacteria, and kill them outright" (*The Green Tea Book*, Lester A. Mitscher, PhD).

# Miso Drink

Here is a warm, healthy and cleansing drink full of protein. It can accompany a meal in the same way as a broth, or drink it as a snack. It is the simplest way of using miso.

O   suitable                          B    not suitable

A   suitable                          AB   suitable

I CUP

I tbsp miso .                         I cup hot water (just below boiling point)

1.   Place the tablespoon of miso in a bowl or mug. Add a little water to dilute the miso then add the remaining water. Drink warm.

## Ingredient Info: Miso

For information on miso see the Miso Soup recipe on page 55.

# super vegetable and fruit juice

Juicing is an excellent way of providing your body with extra vitality. Juices are a rich source of vitamins, minerals, phytonutrients and enzymes. The enzyme content is particularly important as enzymes are only to be found in food that has not been heated. Considered to be the spark of life, the "magic" in our cells, enzymes enable chemical reactions to occur. Life is not possible without them and life is of a better quality when they are plentiful in your diet. For more information on enzymes read the excellent book by Dr Anthony Cichoke *The Complete Book of Enzyme Therapy.*

Compared to supplements, vegetable juices give additional nutrients – some of which have not yet been identified. By breaking down the fibre the nutrients become more easily available to the body. Juicing has been used therapeutically for the past century to heal many conditions. For instance, Dr Max Gerson is well known for his cancer cure based on juices.

How much juice can you drink? This depends on what you wish to achieve. Between one and three glasses a day is roughly equivalent to supplementing your diet with extra nutrients. If you wish to treat a disease you may need to drink between 1 and 8 pints a day. If you are doing a juice fast you will need to be medically supervised.

Virtually all vegetables and fruits can be put through a juicer with the exception of bananas and avocados. Some need peeling such as kiwis, papayas, oranges and grapefruit. Just remove the orange and yellow thin skin of the latter, leaving the white pith. This is rich in bioflavonoids that are valuable for strengthening the capillaries. You may also leave the seeds with the exception of apple seeds. They contain minute amounts of cyanide. Don't worry if you forget to remove them – this is just a precaution as the amount is really very small.

Some leaves need to be discarded, such as carrot tops. The darker celery leaves can be bitter so you may prefer to remove these, though from a health point of view they are very valuable. Drink your juice as soon as you have made it to get the full benefit of the freshness.

# Super Vegetable Juice for Group O

This juice is good for all blood groups but it is specially good for blood group O. It is a good base for adding other vegetables and herbs. Serve it half way through the day or between meals.

| BIG GLASS

3 carrots, unpeeled
1 medium beetroot (beet), unpeeled
5 broccoli florets

½ non-treated lemon with peel
½ inch/1cm cube fresh ginger root

1. Use organic vegetables if possible. Wash and scrub the vegetables. Cut them into pieces small enough to be run through the juicer.
2. Juice all the vegetables and drink immediately.

# Super Vegetable Juice for Group A

**This juice is good for all blood groups but it is specially good for blood group A. It is a good base for adding other vegetables and herbs. This juice makes an excellent snack or light lunch.**

3 carrots, unpeeled
1 medium beetroot (beet), unpeeled
1 celery stalk

½ fennel bulb
½ non-treated lemon, with peel
½ inch/1cm cube fresh ginger root with peel

1.  Use organic vegetables if possible. Wash and scrub the vegetables. Cut them into pieces small enough to be run through the juicer.
2.  Juice all vegetables and drink immediately.

## Ingredient Info: Celery

Celery was first used as a medicinal remedy before being cultivated as a food. It is an excellent source of the minerals potassium, sodium and chloride. Proper muscle contraction and nerve transmission depend on a good balance of these minerals. They also determine water balance in the body.

Celery is traditionally used as a diuretic to balance water distribution in the body, as a slimming aid, nerve tonic, and for lack of appetite, slow digestion, and to treat arthritis, impotence, and various skin problems. The Indian naturopath H. K. Bakhru, reports: "Celery is known to have antispasmodic properties and is useful in the treatment of asthma, bronchitis …" He also states that celery is useful in cases of gall bladder and kidney stones and in the prevention of these disorders.

Science has also uncovered some interesting facts. Celery has been shown to contribute significantly to lowering blood pressure. A researcher at the University of Chicago found that celery contained a blood pressure lowering agent. His research was initiated by a real life experience reported by the father of one of the researchers. He was advised to eat 2 stalks of celery each day for a week. In this short time his blood pressure fell from a high 158/96 to a normal 118/82.

Celery also contains a host of anti-cancer compounds. It seems that the beneficial effects of celery are in the phytonutrients and essential oils rather than in the nutrient content.

# Super Vegetable Juice for Group B

This juice is good for all blood groups but it is specially good for blood group B. It is a good base for adding other vegetables and herbs. This juice is excellent as part of lunch or as a snack instead of fruit.

I BIG GLASS

3 carrots, unpeeled

I medium beetroot (beet), unpeeled

I piece of cauliflower the size of a lemon or 5
 broccoli florets

½ non-treated lemon with peel

½ inch/ I cm cube fresh ginger root

1. Use organic vegetables if possible. Wash and scrub the vegetables. Cut them into pieces small enough to be run through the juicer.
2. Juice all the vegetables and drink immediately.

# Super Vegetable Juice for Group AB

This juice is good for all blood groups but it is specially good for blood group AB. It is a good base for adding other vegetables and herbs. If you're a fan of soup try this instead; it's especially good during the summer months when most people don't feel like having hot soups.

I BIG GLASS

3 carrots, unpeeled

I medium beetroot (beet), unpeeled

I celery stalk

I piece of cauliflower the size of a lemon or 5
 broccoli florets

½ non-treated lemon with peel

½ inch/ I cm cube fresh ginger root

1. Use organic vegetables if possible. Wash and scrub the vegetables. Cut them into pieces small enough to be run through the juicer.
2. Juice all vegetables and drink immediately.

# festive cakes

Cakes are associated with festivities: birthdays, weddings, anniversaries, family events and gatherings. There is something special about cutting a cake that is going to be shared by all those sitting around the same table.

Can we do without cakes? I think not. We can, however, make the best out of this custom by reserving their consumption for these occasions. (Read the text on sugar on pages 145–146 to discover exactly why we need to limit our intake). If you make your own cakes you will eat them less often. It is so easy to buy a cake, whereas it takes more time to make one.

We have included three cakes in this section. The Three Ginger Cake makes use of fresh, ground and candied ginger. The Williamsburg Cake has a wonderful orange and walnut flavour. The Festive Cake is quite elaborate and consists of three thin layers of a spongy cake dough with two different fillings and a lemon-flavoured icing. This cake was extended (multiplied by 6) to make a wedding cake for 120 people. We have given you our tricks if you wish to experience this adventure – wedding cakes are often not the best part of the meal, but this is one people will remember.

# Our Festive Cake

This exquisite and very special cake has evolved over the years from recipes of different countries. It consists of three layers of a light breadcrumb cake dough, filled with one layer of plum purée, one layer of a rich coffee and butter cream, and topped with a very lemony icing. The contrast in taste of the two different layers and the topping give the cake its unusual character. Bake and finish the cake at least two days in advance – it will then be moist with intermingled flavours.

| | | |
|---|---|---|
| O | not suitable | This cake can be enjoyed by Type Bs only. |
| A | not suitable | However, we feel that cakes are part of life's |
| B | suitable | festivities and can be enjoyed by all occasionally at |
| AB | not suitable | special events. |

20 SERVINGS

---

4½lb/2kg pitted dark red plums, fresh or frozen
1 cup/100g fine breadcrumbs made from ½
    white baguette dried in the oven
1¼ cup/230g white sugar
7 organic eggs at room temperature, yolks and
    whites separated
Juice and finely grated zest of 1 non-treated
    lemon
1 tsp ground cinnamon
1 cup/100g finely ground blanched almonds
1 tsp vanilla extract
1 pinch salt

4 tbsp good quality instant coffee
4 tbsp vodka
¾ cup/150g caster (superfine) sugar
¾lb/350g unsalted butter, at room temperature
4–5 tbsp Kirsch (pear, raspberry, or plum
    eau-de-vie)
Juice of 1 lemon
1 cup/150g icing (confectioner's) sugar
Juice of 1 lemon
2½ cups/250g icing (confectioner's) sugar
20 walnut halves to decorate the cake

1. Cook the plum purée a day in advance. In a large cast iron casserole, bring the plums to the boil, reduce the heat and simmer until you get a well cooked, thick mass. Process the plums to a purée in a food processor or blender then leave to cool. The purée should be thick enough to spread with a wide knife or metal spatula without dripping down on the sides of the cake. Check the purée when it has cooled and if you feel it is still too liquid, simmer again to evaporate the moisture. The plums should have the consistency of thick mashed potatoes. Set aside.
2. Cut the baguette into thin slices. Place in a slow warm oven until the bread becomes dry and crisp but not brown. Allow it to cool then grind in a food processor.
3. Line three rectangular cake tins (pans) 9 x 13 in/22 x 33cm with greaseproof (waxed) paper. Preheat the oven to 190°C/375°F/Gas mark 5.

4.  Now prepare the cake. Whip the sugar and the egg yolks until you obtain a light, frothy mixture. Add the lemon zest, lemon juice, cinnamon, ground almonds, breadcrumbs and vanilla. Mix well.

5.  Whip the egg whites with a pinch of salt until they are stiff and keep their shape but not until they are dry. Gently fold a little of the whites into the breadcrumb mixture, then fold in the rest. Divide the dough equally between the three cake tins (pans). Allow the dough to spread over the surface and into the corners by gently tilting the cake tin (pan). Finish off by using a spatula to even off the surface. Bake in the oven for 15–20 minutes or until lightly golden. Set aside to cool.

6.  While the cake is cooling, make the coffee butter. Dissolve the coffee in the vodka. If the vodka comes straight out of the freezer, warm it up before adding to the coffee. Add the sugar to the butter and stir well until the mixture becomes light. Add the coffee mixture and mix well until all the butter is integrated.

7.  Now assemble the cake. Place the first cake layer on a work surface and, with the aid of a spatula, spread the plum purée on the cake and well into the cake corners.

8.  Place the second layer of cake over the plum purée and gently press down. Sprinkle 4–5 tablespoons of Kirsch or other "eau-de-vie" on the cake. Spread the coffee butter evenly on the cake. Place the third layer on the cake (topside on the top), and press lightly.

9.  Now coat the top of the cake with a preliminary icing – we have found that the preliminary icing allows a very neat final icing. Mix the juice of 1 lemon with 1 cup/150g of icing (confectioner's) sugar. Spread a thin coat of this icing over the top of the cake. Set aside to dry.

10. For the final icing, mix the juice of 1 lemon with 2½ cups of icing (confectioner's) sugar. Spread evenly over the top of the cake.

11. Finish off by decorating the cake with the 20 walnut halves. We placed them in rows on the cake so that each cut piece would have a walnut half. Refrigerate for 2–3 days, well covered. After this time the alcohol will have evaporated and only the taste will remain.

# Three Ginger Cake

This cake was inspired by one seen many years ago in a gourmet magazine. We changed the ingredients and quantities to make this deliciously healthy treat.

O    suitable

A    suitable

B    omit the cinnamon

AB   suitable

8–10 SERVINGS

½ cup/200g brown sugar

1 cup/250ml olive oil

1 cup/250ml molasses

½ cup/125ml water

2 eggs, lightly beaten

1 tbsp grated fresh ginger root

3 cups/420g white spelt flour – reserve 1 tbsp

1 tbsp ground cinnamon

2 tsp bicarbonate of soda (baking soda)

1½ tsp ground cloves

1 tbsp ground ginger

1 pinch sea salt

1 cup/150g chopped candied ginger

1.  Preheat the oven to 180°C/350°F/Gas mark 4.
2.  Oil and flour a 10 inch/25cm cake tin (pan).
3.  Combine the brown sugar, olive oil, molasses, water, eggs, and fresh ginger in a large mixing bowl.
4.  Sift the flour, cinnamon, bicarbonate of soda (baking soda), cloves, ground ginger and salt.
5.  Stir the sifted dry ingredients into the wet ingredients, mixing thoroughly.
6.  Mix the candied ginger with the reserved tablespoon of flour and mix into the cake batter.
7.  Pour the mixture into the prepared cake tin (pan) and bake for about 60–70 minutes, until the tester comes out clean. Turn the cake upside down on a wire rack to cool before removing the tin (pan).

## Ingredient Info: Ginger

Ginger has been used in India and China as a food and a medicine since ancient times. Its versatility in cooking is almost endless. It can be used with fish, meat, fowl, vegetables, fruit, legumes; you can drink it as a tea, and eat it as a dessert (candied ginger).

Its uses as a medicine are also numerous. Ginger is very beneficial for a variety of digestive disorders: flatulence, spasms, vomiting, nausea, travel and morning sickness, stomach aches, diarrhoea and constipation. In Ayurvedic medicine it is thought to strengthen the digestion.

Inflammatory conditions accompanied by pain, such as rheumatoid arthritis and migraine, will benefit from the regular intake of ginger. In this case the ground ginger in capsule form is usually recommended. Ginger is also good for the circulatory system. It contains active substances that inhibit blood clotting and it promotes blood circulation, specially to the hands and feet.

If you feel a cold coming on try drinking ginger tea: add 4 or 5 slices of fresh ginger root to a cup of boiling water and allow it to steep for 10 minutes. Drink several cups a day.

For medicinal purposes, ginger is used fresh or dried in powdered form. It can also be juiced and added to freshly extracted vegetable and fruit juices.

Just by adding ginger regularly in your meals you will benefit from its immense health-giving qualities. Anything that strengthens the digestive system will do a world of good to your general well-being.

Also see the information on ginger on page 161.

# valerie's wedding cake

If you feel like setting forth on this cake adventure, do practise making *Our Festive Cake* on page 169 as the wedding cake is simply the same recipe multiplied by six. By increasing the ingredients and following the same method we managed to make a delicious wedding cake for 120 people. It took guts, time, concentration and good organization – as well as a little extra help – but we definitely feel anyone can do the same.

When Karen's daughter announced her forthcoming wedding, we happily offered to make her wedding cake. The ceremony was to take place in Berlin, we were in Paris. The young couple's kitchen would be our cooking ground.

It was obvious that the more we could do in advance, in our respective homes, the easier it would be. So we got together all the bits and pieces we would need – cake tins, gold Kraft paper for presenting the cake etc. etc. – and prepared the plum purée (and froze it) and the fine breadcrumbs in advance.

Then it was off to Berlin by car. Three days before "The Day" we set to work, as the cake needed to be cooked in advance. We started at 11am and finally finished at 10pm, having taken only an hour off for lunch. The "extra help" came in the form of a group of the bride and groom's friends who made themselves very useful by shelling 4 pounds of walnuts in order to obtain 120 perfect halves. We knew through experience that you break a lot of nuts in the shelling process, so you need plenty to get the required amount of perfect halves. Their enthusiasm and effort was much appreciated.

For 120 people we made six cakes using the recipe for *Our Festive Cake*. Each of these cakes serves 20 people. First of all we started off making 18 cake layers, followed by six times the coffee butter. Once all of this was done we started assembling each cake one by one on greaseproof (waxed) paper. A thick coating of plum purée was placed on the first layer of cake. Next came the second cake layer, sprinkled with some *eau de vie* and a thick coating of coffee butter. Finally we added the third layer of cake with its thin coating of preliminary icing. Each cake was then covered with greaseproof (waxed) paper, then aluminium foil. The six cakes were then placed in the refrigerator for two days – it was the 23rd of June and Berlin was hot.

We decided to assemble the cake and do the final icing on the wedding day as we didn't have anywhere big enough to refrigerate it. We bought a thick, square piece of plywood 2ft 10in/86cm – having previously checked if it would fit horizontally through the kitchen door and then in the trunk of the car – and covered this with gold Kraft paper. First of all we stuck the paper to the plywood with a thin coat of preliminary icing. This was essential for the transportation, as the weight of the cake could have ripped the paper from the wood if there had been an abrupt stop.

Once all the cakes were side by side on the gold paper, we filled in the space left around the corners with the broken pieces of walnuts. Then came the thick white icing over the thin preliminary icing and over all the cakes. A perfectly white shining mirror appeared. On each cake we placed 20 perfect walnut halves. Not only did they serve as decoration but also they helped determine where to cut the cake. To strengthen the sides of the cake we first of all put a hard transparent border around it (bought at a wholesale pastry shop) and finished off with 2 inch/5cm thick white satin ribbon, around the cake.

We had planned to decorate the board with white flowers but in the bustle of the whole event had forgotten to order them!

The final result was greatly appreciated by all.

# The Cake

120 PEOPLE

FOR THE CAKE:
3½lb/1.5kg sugar
42 organic eggs
6 non-treated lemons, preferably organic
6 tsp ground cinnamon
6 cups/675g finely ground blanched almonds
6 cups/675g fine breadcrumbs made from 3 white baguettes dried in the oven
6 tsp vanilla extract
6 pinches salt

PLUM PURÉE:
27lb/12kg dark red plums

FOR THE SECOND CAKE LAYER:
2 cups/500ml Kirsch (pear, raspberry or cherry eau-de-vie, 45% or more alcohol)

COFFEE BUTTER:
4½lb/2kg unsalted butter, at room temperature
2lb/900g caster (superfine) sugar
24 tbsp good quality instant coffee
24 tbsp vodka

PRELIMINARY ICING:
Juice of 6 lemons
2lb/900g icing (confectioner's) sugar

FINAL ICING:
Juice of 6 lemons
3½lb/1.5kg icing (confectioner's) sugar

6 rectangular cake tins 9 x 13 inch/22 x 33cm

FOR DECORATION:
120 perfect walnut halves, we bought 4lb/2kg and shelled them
1 thick square plywood board 2'10" x 2'10"/86cm x 86cm (check that the board can go horizontally through both kitchen and house doors)
1 roll gold Kraft paper (bought at a wholesale store for pastry shops)
5 yards/5 metres hard transparent pastry border to protect the sides of the cake and also the white satin ribbon
5 yards/5 metres white satin ribbon
White flowers to decorate

# Williamsburg Cake

This is our version of the traditional Williamsburg cake, which we discovered many years ago. Ever since, it has graced our tables as the family's favourite birthday cake. It is all the better made 1 or 2 days in advance.

| | | |
|---|---|---|
| O | not suitable | Strictly speaking this cake may be eaten by Bs only. |
| A | not suitable | As and ABs should avoid butter and buttermilk |
| B | suitable | whereas Os should avoid buttermilk. However, we |
| AB | not suitable | feel that cakes are part of life's festivities and can be |
| | | enjoyed by all occasionally. |

8–10 SERVINGS

2 organic oranges

1½ cups/215g sifted white spelt flour

½ tsp sea salt

1 tsp bicarbonate of soda (baking soda)

1 cup dark seedless raisins, roughly chopped

¾ cup/150g chopped walnuts or pecans

¾ cup/150g brown sugar

½ cup/100g unsalted butter, at room temperature

2 large organic eggs

1 cup/250ml buttermilk

1 tsp vanilla extract

ICING:

2 cups icing (confectioner's) sugar

5 tbsp/75g unsalted butter, at room temperature

3–4 tsp dry sherry

1 large egg white

1 segment orange peel, very finely chopped

1. Preheat the oven to 190°C/375° F/Gas mark 5. Butter and flour a 10 inch/25cm cake tin (pan).
2. Score each orange into 4 segments, peel them and set aside 1 segment.
3. Mix the flour, salt, baking soda, raisins and nuts in a mixing bowl and set aside.
4. Mince the 7 orange peel segments with half the sugar in the food processor until the orange peel is reduced to small specks. Add to the flour mixture.
5. Mix the softened butter with the rest of the sugar until smooth. Add the eggs one by one, then the buttermilk and the vanilla. The mixture should not be overly mixed. Add the flour mixture and the sugar/orange peel mixture until the flour just disappears. Do not mix too thoroughly.
6. Pour the batter into the floured tin (pan) and bake for 30–35 minutes or until a knife comes out clean.
7. Allow the cake to cool completely on a wire rack before icing.
8. Now prepare the icing. Mix all the icing ingredients, except the orange peel, with a small wire whisk until smooth. Add the finely chopped orange peel and, with a spatula, spread the icing on the cake. Wait at least a day before eating.

# christmas recipes

Christmas is a time for getting together and enjoying a treat or two, so it's nice to be able to pull out some home-baked biscuits or a slice of Christmas cake that you have made yourself.

The Christmas cakes and biscuits featured in this section make big use of nuts and dried fruits and little use of sugar (see pages 145–146 on the drawbacks of sugar). The Christmas Fruit Cake has evolved out of 25 years of baking it every year for our Christmas festivities, so it has stood the test of time. Our Christmas biscuits are similar to those traditionally baked in the Germanic and Scandinavian countries. They are usually baked several weeks in advance as this improves their taste. However, you must store them in separate air-tight boxes for them to retain their texture.

# Almond and Raisin Biscuits (Cookies)

These Christmas biscuits (cookies) are adapted from a traditional Swiss recipe. Make them 3–4 weeks in advance – this improves their taste – and keep them in their own air-tight box. You will only need the yolks of the eggs for this recipe, but you can use up the whites for the other Christmas recipes.

O  suitable             B  suitable

A  not suitable        AB  not suitable

MAKES 90

| | |
|---|---|
| 1 cup/225g butter | 3¼ cups/400g white spelt flour |
| Generous ½ cup/115g brown sugar | 1¼ cups/100g slivered almonds |
| 4 egg yolks | ¾ cup/100g small raisins |

1. Mix the butter and sugar until it reaches a creamy consistency. Add the egg yolks and flour. Knead the mixture until it forms a dough.
2. Divide the dough into 2 equal parts.
3. Add the raisins to one half of the dough and the almonds to the other half. Persistent kneading will help incorporate these ingredients.
4. Make each half into a roll 1½ inches/4cm thick. Wrap in greaseproof (waxed) paper and place overnight in the refrigerator.
5. Before cooking preheat the oven to 200°C/400°F/Gas mark 6.
6. With a sharp, thin knife cut your roll into rounds ¼ inch/5mm thick.
7. Place the biscuits (cookies) on baking sheets lined with greaseproof (waxed) paper. Bake 8–10 minutes until lightly golden.

# Christmas Fruit Cake

This version of a fruit cake needs to be made at least one month in advance for it to acquire the rich, dense and mellow taste from the blending of the varied ingredients. It is densely packed with dried fruit and improves with age, so avoid the temptation to eat it before its time.

O  replace nutmeg with allspice

A  not suitable

B  suitable

AB  not suitable

2 CAKES

1½ cups/250g pitted dates

1¼ cups/200g dried figs

1 cup/160g dried apricots

1¼ cups/120g walnuts, broken into pieces

1 cup/160g Malaga or other dark raisins

1 cup/160g currants

1 cup/160g sultanas (white raisins)

1 cup/140g spelt flour

1 cup/200g butter

1 cup/ 200g brown sugar

4 organic eggs

2 cups/280g spelt flour

1 tsp baking powder

1 tsp sea salt

4 tsp ground cinnamon

1 tsp ground nutmeg

½ cup/125ml red grape juice

1 tsp vanilla extract

1 cup/250ml bourbon

1. Preheat the oven to 140°C/275°F/Gas mark 1. Butter two 10 x 3¾ inch/25 x 9.5cm cake tins (pans) and line with buttered greaseproof (waxed) paper.
2. Chop the dates, figs and apricots into pieces slightly less than ½ inch/1cm. Mix in the walnuts, raisins, currants and sultanas (white raisins). Add the 1 cup/140g flour to the fruit and nut mixture. Set aside.
3. Beat the butter with the sugar until fluffy. Beat in the eggs one by one. Set aside.
4. Mix the 2 cups/280g flour, baking powder, salt and spices together in a large bowl.
5. Blend the butter mixture gradually with the flour and spice mixture, adding the fruit juice and vanilla extract as you go.
6. Pour this over the fruit and nuts and mix thoroughly. Fill the cake tins (pans) with the mixture and bake in the oven for 2½–3 hours. The cakes mustn't become too dark on the top. If they begin to brown too quickly, place a piece of foil over the top. Let the cakes cool completely before turning them out.
7. Use soft white cotton muslin to wrap the cakes. Pour about ¼ cup/60ml bourbon on a plate and soak the pieces of fabric. Wring them out and wrap around each cake. Cover with foil and keep the cakes in a closed container in a cool place. After a few days check the dryness of the cloth and renew the bourbon procedure as often as necessary until Christmas. Two days before eating the cake remove the cloth, replace with greaseproof (waxed) paper and cover again with foil. Keep in the refrigerator until serving.

# Hazelnut Leckerli

As with the other two Christmas biscuit (cookie) recipes, make these 3–4 weeks in advance and keep them in their own air-tight box. The leckerli, as well as the Cinnamon Stars, can be made with the egg whites left over from making the Almond and Raisin Biscuits.

O suitable

A suitable

B not suitable

AB not suitable

MAKES 78

¾lb/340g roasted hazelnuts with their skins (see instructions page 194)

½lb/225g hazelnuts with their skins

½lb/225g almonds with their skins

2 cups/300g brown sugar

¼lb/115 g candied orange peel, finely diced

Zest of 2 non-treated lemons

1 cup/150g mild tasting honey

2 tbsp Kirsch

2 egg whites, whipped until they form stiff peaks

1 cup/150g hazelnuts for decoration

1. Grind the roasted and unroasted hazelnuts and the almonds in a food processor until they reach the consistency of coarse crystallized sugar. Transfer to a large mixing bowl.
2. Add the sugar, orange peel, lemon zest, honey, Kirsch and lastly the whipped egg whites. Stir with a wooden spoon until all the ingredients are well incorporated. Knead with the palm of your hands until the dough holds in a ball. (Kneading encourages the extraction of the nut oils.)
3. Moisten the surface on which you will be working. Take some of the dough, flatten it down and with a wet palm pat it to a thickness of a ½ inch/1cm.
4. Wet a 1½ inch/4cm cookie cutter and cut out your leckerli. Occasionally you will need to wash the cutter so that it makes clean cuts. Place each leckerli on a baking sheet covered with greaseproof (waxed) paper.
5. Once all the leckerlis are cut out, decorate the centre of each one with a hazelnut. Let them dry, uncovered, for several hours or overnight at room temperature.
6. Heat the oven to 180°C/350°F/Gas mark 4, and bake the biscuits (cookies) for 10 minutes maximum. When the leckerlis have cooled down they should be soft and springy; if they're hard they have been overcooked.

# Cinnamon Stars

These biscuits (cookies) should be made 3–4 weeks in advance, as their taste improves with time. Keep them separately in their own air-tight box. If you make these at the same time as the Almond and Raisin Biscuits (Cookies), you can use the left-over egg whites from that recipe.

| | | | |
|---|---|---|---|
| O | suitable | B | not suitable |
| A | suitable | AB | suitable |

70 STARS

| | |
|---|---|
| 1lb/450g almonds with their skins | 1 tbsp Kirsch |
| 1½ cups/350g brown sugar | 3 egg whites, whipped until they form stiff peaks |
| 2½ tbsp ground cinnamon, less if you prefer a lighter taste | |

1.  Grind the almonds in a food processor until they reach the consistency of coarse crystallized sugar. Transfer to a large mixing bowl.
2.  Add the sugar, cinnamon, Kirsch and lastly the whipped egg whites. Stir with a wooden spoon until all the ingredients are well incorporated. Knead with the palm of your hand until the dough holds together in a ball. (Kneading encourages the extraction of the almond oil.)
3.  Moisten the surface on which you will be working. Take some of the dough, flatten it and with a wet palm pat it down to a thickness of ¼ inch/5mm.
4.  Wet a 1½ inch/4cm diameter star cutter and start cutting out your stars. You will need to wash the star cutter occasionally so that it makes a perfect star. Place the stars on a baking sheet covered with greaseproof (waxed) paper and sprinkled with a little sugar.
6.  Let the stars dry for several hours or overnight, uncovered, at room temperature.
7.  Heat the oven to 180°C/350°F/Gas mark 4, and bake the stars for 10 minutes maximum. When the stars have cooled down they should be soft and springy; if they're hard they have been overcooked.

## Ingredient Info: Cinnamon

Cinnamon is the ground inner bark of an evergreen tree native to Sri Lanka and India. It has been used for several thousand years, both medicinally and in cooking. The Chinese, Romans, and Egyptians knew of its medicinal virtues. Today cinnamon is still regularly used in China and India for healing.

Cinnamon is good for preventing colds and can also help to ease the effects of one. Mix a drink of warm water, ¼–½ teaspoon of ground cinnamon and ginger, the juice and zest of half a lemon, and a teaspoonful of honey if the taste is too pungent for you. Take small sips at a time. Cinnamon is known as a warming spice so it can make you sweat.

Cinnamon also has well known digestive properties. It counteracts nausea, vomiting and diarrhoea and improves digestion in general. It has a sedative and antispasmodic effect on aching muscles.

# basic recipes

Throughout our recipes you will need to refer to these basic recipes every now and then. You will discover how to make stock for soups, roast nuts and seeds, prepare clarified butter for cooking, preserve lemons for use in meat and poultry dishes, prepare a marinade for game, make an instant mayonnaise, a thin pie crust to make the fruit pies, and the different methods for soaking beans.

# stock

Stock – whether made from chicken, meat, fish or vegetables – is an invaluable addition to cooking, both in terms of taste and health. Good quality stock is a fundamental part of fine cuisine, adding flavour and depth to sauces and soups.

The Chinese make soups – usually based on chicken broth – that they claim have all sorts of health benefits: they strengthen the immune system, enhance blood circulation, raise your energy levels and protect against cancer. You may have heard your grandmother recommend chicken broth at the first signs of a cold. Research has shown chicken soup to be effective against the common cold. It is an old remedy well known to the Jewish culture. Meat and fish broth contain valuable minerals such as calcium, magnesium and potassium and other elements found in cartilage that are good for bones and joints. Research has shown that rheumatoid arthritis sufferers given collagen from chicken cartilage experienced relief after three months.

Freshly made stock is a liquid full of still-unknown properties, but its positive effects on health have been well known for centuries, and have now been confirmed by modern research. It is well worth including stock in your cooking repertoire – it takes little effort and adds immense value to a whole range of dishes.

Once you have cooked your stock, cool it quickly by setting the stock pot in cold water. Transfer to the refrigerator and the next day remove the fat that will have risen to the top. Precautions must be taken for keeping stock as it has a tendency to easily ferment. You may keep poultry and vegetable stock for three days in the refrigerator, and fish stock for two days. Boil before using. Stock can also be frozen for future use.

# Chicken or Turkey Stock

**This stock is good enough to be eaten as a soup. As a stock it will enhance all your dishes. Do ensure, however, that you use free-range poultry.**

O   use chicken or turkey

A   use chicken or turkey; omit the peppercorns

B   use turkey

AB  use turkey; omit the peppercorns

---

1 large free-range chicken or small turkey or
    2–3lb/1–1.5kg of chicken or turkey pieces
2 medium onions, roughly chopped
4 celery stalks, roughly chopped
4 tbsp freshly squeezed lemon juice
6 garlic cloves, unpeeled

2 bay leaves
3 sprigs of thyme
10 black peppercorns
Sea salt
3¾ quarts/4 litres cold filtered water

1. Place all the ingredients in a stainless steel stock pot and cover with the water. Bring to the boil, removing any impurities that rise to the surface, lower the heat and simmer for 2–3 hours.
2. Strain the stock through a fine sieve into a large container and place in cold water to cool. This procedure protects the stock from developing bacteria, which multiply quickly in this warm medium. Refrigerate only when the stock is cold. The following day remove the solidified fat. This stock will keep for three days; boil before using. You may also freeze the stock in glass containers without their tops, cover once frozen.

# Fish Stock

**Fish stock is the basis of all fish soups. Use it as it is or add a dash of dry white wine, fresh coriander (cilantro) leaves, sticks of fresh ginger root and a few drops of freshly squeezed lemon juice. When making your stock, only use lean fish that are recommended for your blood group.**

O  suitable

A  omit the peppercorns

B  suitable

AB  omit the peppercorns

---

I tbsp extra virgin olive oil
I medium onion, finely chopped
I shallot, finely chopped
3 celery stalks
Parsley stalks

3lb/1.5kg heads and bones from lean fish
1½ quarts/1½ litres fresh filtered water
I bouquet garni – thyme, bay leaf etc.
Juice of ½ lemon
Sea salt and black peppercorns

1. Heat the olive oil in a large stock pot. Add the vegetables and let them sweat for 5 minutes without allowing them to brown. During this time remove gills from fish heads and rinse the bones and heads under running water. Roughly chop the fish bones and add to the vegetables. Let all the ingredients sweat for another 5 minutes. Add the cold water, bouquet garni, lemon juice and seasoning. Bring to the boil, lower the heat and simmer for 20 minutes. Skim any impurities that rise to the top.

2. Let the stock set for 15 minutes and ladle it through a fine-meshed sieve, leaving the impurities at the bottom of the stockpot. If you wish, you may now reduce the stock over very low heat to concentrate it further. This stock can be kept for a maximum of two days in the refrigerator or freeze it for up to three months.

# Vegetable Stock

This vegetable stock can be varied according to the season. In winter use celery root, swiss chard, winter squashes etc. In the summer use courgettes (zucchini), fennel, tomatoes, etc., and basil, marjoram and oregano as herbs. Certain vegetables – broccoli, cauliflower, Brussels sprouts, cabbage and turnips – are best avoided as they can give off a strong unpleasant taste.

| O | omit the leeks | B | suitable |
|---|---|---|---|
| A | omit the peppercorns | AB | omit the peppercorns |

---

2 tbsp olive oil
1 large onion, roughly chopped
3 large leeks, roughly chopped
2 medium carrots, roughly chopped
3 celery stalks, with leaves roughly chopped
6 crushed garlic cloves with their skins
1 tsp sea salt

6 parsley sprigs or stems
2 bay leaves
4 fresh thyme sprigs or ½ tsp dried thyme
4 fresh sage leaves or a pinch of dried leaves
1 tsp whole peppercorns
2 quarts/2 litres cold filtered water

1. Heat the oil in a stainless steel stock pot. Add all the vegetables, including the garlic, then the salt. Stir the vegetables over a low heat for 10 minutes. Add the herbs and water and simmer for 1½ hours or more.
2. Strain through a sieve, pressing the vegetables to extract as much liquid as possible. Either use the stock immediately or let it cool before refrigerating or freezing. Discard the vegetables.

# Clarified Butter

The process of clarifying butter removes the milk protein, leaving pure fat. Clarified butter can therefore be tolerated by those sensitive to milk products. It is also excellent for cooking as it doesn't burn and therefore will not produce harmful carcinogenic substances. Clarifying butter also eliminates lectins. The best cooking fats are olive oil and clarified butter as they are the least sensitive to heat treatment. Avoid using other cold pressed oils for cooking as their molecular structure makes them sensitive to heat and harmful to health when heated. Ordinary butter can be used but clarified butter is better. Always choose organic butter as pesticides tend to concentrate in the fatty portion of milk. Clarified butter has a delicious nutty flavour. It can be used in many ways: for frying, to put on vegetables before serving, on bread instead of butter, in the ingredients of your fruit crumble topping ...

| | | | |
|---|---|---|---|
| O | suitable | B | suitable |
| A | suitable | AB | suitable |

---

2lb/1kg unsalted organic butter, cut into small
    pieces

1. Melt the butter in a heavy saucepan over low heat. Let it simmer very gently for 10–30 minutes. The cooking time will depend on the amount of water in the butter. Quite rapidly you will see a white froth appear on the surface of the melted liquid. Remove this with a slotted spoon. The leftover solid particles from the milk will drop to the bottom and/or stick to the sides of the pan. Eventually they will take on a golden colour. Keep watching as this phenomena indicates that the butter is clarified. The liquid butter becomes almost transparent.

2. When the butter reaches this stage, very carefully pour the liquid through a muslin cloth or a fine handkerchief into an earthenware jar, leaving the golden particles at the bottom. Clarified butter can be stored at room temperature or in the refrigerator for several weeks. As there are no more milk solids, it does not have to be refrigerated.

# preparing dried beans

There are two ways of preparing beans for cooking – one is quick, the other a little more lengthy. Do bear in mind, however, that the more you soak and rinse beans the less gas they produce.

## Method 1: The long cold soak

Soak the beans in a large amount of water overnight. Pour off the soaking water and rinse. Put the beans into a saucepan and cover with water. Cook them for 5 minutes, skimming off the foam as they cook. Drain and rinse the beans again and cover with fresh water. Now cook the beans for the time specified on the packet.

## Method 2: The quick hot soak

This second method is great if you have forgotten to soak your beans overnight and still want to eat them. Bring the beans to the boil in a pot of cold water and let them cook for 3 minutes. Turn off the heat and leave them to soak for one hour. Pour off the soaking water, rinse the beans and cover them with fresh water. Now cook the beans for the time specified on the packet.

Adding a seaweed called kombu can help make the beans more digestible. Garlic, ginger, herbs and spices in general are traditionally added to beans to avoid excessive gas production. Only add salt and acid foods such as tomatoes towards the end of the cooking time as this could otherwise harden the outside skin and make cooking more difficult.

# Marinade for Game

This marinade can be used with boar, venison and other big game. Type As – who should avoid game – can use this marinade for ostrich meat or chicken.

| O | suitable | B | suitable |
|---|----------|---|----------|
| A | suitable | AB | suitable |

---

3 cups/750ml red wine

1 carrot, cut into slices

1 onion, cut into fine slices

5 garlic cloves, unpeeled

Thyme, rosemary and bay leaf

10 juniper berries

Zest of ½ organic orange

3 tbsp olive oil

1. Bring the wine to the boiling stage. Add the remaining ingredients, with the exception of the olive oil, and cook at low temperature for 30 minutes. Allow it to cool, then add the olive oil and mix well.
2. Place the meat to be marinated in an earthenware dish, pour the marinade over the meat and cover. Rotate the meat twice a day for 1–2 days. It will then be ready for cooking.

# Mayonnaise

**This recipe is made with an electric hand-held blender. Plan ahead and remove any ingredients that are kept in the refrigerator so they are at room temperature when you start. If you follow the step-by-step instructions carefully it will take only a few seconds to produce a successful mayonnaise.**

O   use apple cider vinegar or lemon juice and
vinegar-free mustard

A   use lemon juice and vinegar-free mustard; omit
the pepper

B   suitable

AB   use lemon juice and vinegar-free mustard; omit
the pepper

---

1 organic egg, extra fresh
1 tsp mustard, Dijon if possible
1 pinch sea salt
Freshly ground black pepper
1 tsp red wine vinegar, cider vinegar or lemon
juice

1 cup/250ml olive oil or the oil of your choice

FINISHING TOUCH:
1 tsp vinegar or lemon juice

*All the ingredients must be at room temperature*

1. If your blender does not have its own jar then use one that is a little wider than the base of the blender. Place the egg, then the mustard, salt, pepper, vinegar and finally the oil in the jar.
2. Carefully insert the blender until it reaches the bottom of the jar. Now turn it on and slowly bring it up to the top to incorporate all the oil. The mayonnaise is done.
3. Now add the last teaspoon of vinegar or lemon juice – more if you like the taste – and adjust the seasoning if necessary. This mayonnaise can be kept in the refrigerator for several days. Let it reach room temperature before stirring it.

# Preserved Lemons

This North African speciality is traditionally used in fish, chicken, lamb and rabbit dishes called *tagines*. The preserved peel will soften, take on a very mild yet rich flavour and give a deep aroma to your dishes. Suitable for all blood groups, these lemons are a must to have on hand throughout the year.

| O | suitable | B | suitable |
|---|----------|---|----------|
| A | suitable | AB | suitable |

---

| | |
|---|---|
| 8 small ripe organic lemons | Water |
| I cup coarse sea salt | I quart/I litre jar with a spring top |

1. Wash the lemons well. With a sharp knife remove both ends. Holding the lemon, carefully make a cut halfway through the fruit. Turn the lemon over and make another deep cut halfway through the fruit but this time at a 90 degree angle to the first cut. The cutting lines should not meet.
2. Stuff the cut slits of lemons with sea salt. Press each fruit into the jar and let the juices seep out for 24 hours.
3. Now cover the fruit with fresh water, close the jar and store in a cool dark place for at least 1 month. They will keep in the refrigerator for at least one year.

## Ingredient Info: Lemons

Lemons are native to India. They were known to the Romans but their use became more widespread in southern Europe – where they could easily grow – around the twelfth century. The lemon tree is an evergreen and bears its fruit all year round. The whole fruit – skin, pulp, pith and juice can be used. When making vegetable and fruit juices with an extractor make sure you add a piece of whole lemon for its own benefits but also for its antioxidant effect on the juice you are making.

In Spain, lemons are extensively used for their numerous health benefits. Lemon juice, although it has an acid taste, is not acidifying to the body. On the contrary it has an alcalizing effect and as such is a valuable remedy against all sorts of rheumatic conditions. It has a detoxifying and cleansing effect on the body. Lemons are rich in vitamin C and potassium.

Lemons have many curative properties – the following examples are just a few.

If you have a cold coming on drink the juice of one lemon in a cup of hot water several times a day and specially before going to bed.

Lemons are good for strengthening the blood vessel walls. If you have varicose veins or spider veins on the legs, easy bruising or haemorrhoids use the whole fruit in blended fruit mixes. For example you can blend a banana with half of a seedless lemon. The bioflavonoids in the pith are the active ingredient.

To stimulate your appetite and get those gastric juices going, drink a glass of water with lemon juice. It also has other beneficial effects along the digestive tract. It helps dispel intestinal gases, relieves heartburn, improves liver and gall bladder function and promotes bile secretion.

Lemons also have external uses: rub a slice of lemon on blemished skin, use freshly squeezed juice as a lotion twice a week to protect against wrinkles.

Lemons are a very versatile food in the kitchen. They can be used cooked or raw; in sweet or savoury dishes; with fish, chicken, rabbit, lamb and veal; with legumes, vegetables, salads and fruit; in cakes and biscuits. Every part of the lemon has a use. The pith, although it has a bitter taste, should be used for its bioflavonoids and the seeds are effective against intestinal worms.

When you next buy lemons don't just buy one or two, buy a dozen and include them in all these ways in your daily routine.

# Thin Pie Crust

This is our favourite pie crust dough recipe. We roll the dough until it is paper thin; when cooked it then becomes flaky and similar to a French *pâte feuilletée* (puff pastry). You may use it for both sweet and savoury pies.

O   suitable

A   use clarified butter

B   suitable

AB   use clarified butter

MAKES A 10–11 INCH/25–27CM PIE SHELL

½ cup/125g unsalted butter or clarified butter
    (see recipe page 187), at room temperature
1¾ cups/250g sifted white spelt flour

3–4 tbsp cold water
1 pinch salt, optional

1. Cut the butter into small pieces and place in a bowl with the flour and salt. With two knives cut the butter into the dry ingredients, leaving small pieces of butter intact – this will give it the consistency of *feuilletée*.
2. Sprinkle half of the water over the mixture and incorporate with a wooden spoon. Add more of the water until the dough starts sticking together.
3. Using the heel of your hand gather the dough into a ball. Knead it 4 or 5 times. The less you work with it the better. Cover the dough and let it rest for at least 30 minutes in the refrigerator; longer is better.
4. Dust a little flour over the pie tin (pan). Dust your rolling pin with flour and lightly flour the surface you will be working on.
5. Roll the dough from the centre to the sides until you have the right size for your tin (pan). Wrap the dough lightly around the rolling pin to lift it onto the pie tin (pan). It should have an elastic consistency and be able to be handled quite easily. Mould the dough to the pie tin (pan) and cut away the excess dough. Using a fork, make small holes on the bottom of the pie.
6. Now add your filling, be it sweet or salty.

# how to roast nuts and seeds

There are two advantages to lightly roasting nuts and seeds – the process enhances the taste and makes them more digestible. There are two roasting methods, depending on the size of the nuts and seeds.

## Method 1

Walnuts, almonds, hazelnuts, pecans and pumpkin seeds are best roasted under a grill (broiler). Heat the grill (broiler) and roast the nuts or seeds 4–5 inches/10–12cm from the heat for approximately 10 minutes. Keep checking their colour as they burn very easily. A bitter smell announces that they are over roasted.

## Method 2

Pine nuts, sesame and sunflower seeds are best roasted in a dry frying pan (skillet). Heat the pan. Add the seeds and stir constantly until they are lightly roasted. Watch their colour carefully as pine nuts and seeds burn very easily.

# the blood type diet menus

If you are struggling with meal planning these menus should help you get started. We have planned four seasonal menus for each blood type. This will provide guidance on incorporating the fruits and vegetables of each season into your new eating habits. For weekdays – when most of us tend to have a full schedule – light meals are offered. Saturday starts with a super vegetable juice, followed by breakfast; then a light meal and a meal for sharing with friends is given – have these whichever way round suits your day. Sunday's menu includes a family meal with an appetizer, main course with vegetables, and a real "Sunday" dessert. The entries shown in bold are recipes contained in this book.

On rising, all blood types should have a large glass of natural or filtered water to rehydrate the body. Type A and AB should add the juice of half a lemon to the water. This helps clear out the mucous accumulated overnight, for which these two groups have an added sensitivity. It is better to drink water before and after meals instead of drinking with meals as large quantities of liquid tend to dilute the digestive juices, making them less effective at digestion. Limit yourself to a glass of red wine with your meal.

We have discovered that it is far better for many people to eat three light meals and two snacks (one mid-morning, the other in the afternoon) per day, rather than to have one, two or three big meals. Skipping meals is also a bad idea. The resulting hunger is perceived as stress by the body and is an invitation to drink coffee and tea, which raise blood sugar levels – irrespective of whether or not you add sugar. Avoid falling into the "coffee, croissant or cookie" trap. There is so much out there which provides energy *and* good health. Make a habit of reading labels on food packaging to discover hidden ingredients.

# snacks

Snacks are not incorporated in the menus. Instead a list of what is appropriate for each blood type is given to allow you to choose for yourself. These are only suggestions, however, so add to the list anything that is appropriate for your blood type. Plan your snacks ahead of time so you don't hit the sugar because you need a quick fix. Try to eat your snack at a regular time and before you become ravenous.

We feel the best snacks are fresh and dried fruits, accompanied by nuts and seeds or another form of protein that is suitable for your blood type. The combination of carbohydrate (in the form of fruit) and protein will work to stabilize blood sugar levels. Herbal tea, green tea or our green tea with ginger make healthy drinks.

## Snacks for Os

- In the summer enjoy cherries, raspberries, blueberries, peaches, plums and pears with a protein source such as soya yogurt, goat's or sheep's cheese (the latter every now and then, if you tolerate it).
- For a good winter snack try dried figs, dates, apricots and prunes with walnuts, almonds, hazelnuts, macadamia nuts and pumpkin seeds.
- Bananas, guavas and mangoes are very good for this blood type and can be accompanied by a glass of soya milk.

## Snacks for As

- Apples, apricots, berries, cherries, figs, pears, and all the plums go well with a glass of soya milk or a soya yogurt.
- Dried figs, dates, prunes, apricots, pineapple, raisins, cranberries and apples with a protein source such as pumpkin seeds, walnuts, peanuts, almonds, macadamia nuts, pecans and sunflower seeds make a good snack when the fresh summer fruit has gone.
- Rye crisp crackers, oat and rice cakes spread with peanut butter, sesame paste, almond butter or a tofu spread are good when something more substantial is needed.

## Snacks for Bs

- Enjoy oranges (you are the only one), grapes, berries, and just about all the fruits with a yogurt.
- Dried figs, dates, cranberries, pineapple, banana, raisins and prunes with a protein source such as brazil nuts, walnuts, pecan, macadamia, and almonds make a sustaining snack.
- You are the lucky one who can eat milk products. Have a piece of cheese on a slice of spelt bread or an oat or rice cake. Alternatively, have a glass of milk and a banana or some dates.

## Snacks for ABs

- Enjoy cherries, cranberries, grapes, plums, currants, peaches, apricots, raspberries with sheep's or goat's yogurt.
- Dried figs, apricots, dates, raisins, pineapple, prunes with peanuts, walnuts and almonds make a nutritious snack. You may also have your dried fruits with a glass of soya milk or a soya yogurt.
- Peanut butter or a slice of cheese on a rye cracker, rice cake or Essene bread is good when you need something sustaining.

# spring blood type o

## monday

**Breakfast**

½ grapefruit
1 slice Essene bread with goat's cheese
**Green Tea with Ginger**

**Lunch**

**Broccoli Velouté**
**Tofu Salad**
Dates, figs and walnuts
Peppermint tea

**Dinner**

Steamed fish with **Parsley Sauce**
**Spinach with Currants and Pine Nuts**
Pear

## tuesday

**Breakfast**

1 slice pineapple
Banana with soya milk, ground
    flaxseeds and pumpkin seeds
Peppermint tea

**Lunch**

**Raw Beetroot Salad**
Grilled (broiled) lamb chops
**Broccoli with Ginger and Garlic**

**Dinner**

**Miso Soup**
Grilled (broiled) duck leg with
    **Courgette Purée**
Prunes

## wednesday

**Breakfast**

½ slice mango
1 scrambled egg
1 slice spelt bread, toasted
Dandelion coffee with soya milk

**Lunch**

**Fennel Salad**
**Grilled Tuna** with its sauce
Oven-baked tomatoes
Sheep's yogurt

**Dinner**

Fresh asparagus
**Guinea Fowl with Sage**
Sweet potato
1 slice pineapple

## thursday

**Breakfast**

½ grapefruit
1 slice Essene bread with tahini and
    ½ teaspoon honey
1 soya yogurt
Rose hip tea

**Lunch**

Endive, apple and walnut salad
Calves' liver
Green beans

**Dinner**

**Spinach Salad**
**Goat's Cheese Dumplings**
½ mango

# friday

### Breakfast

1 bowl of cherries
Soya yogurt with 2 figs, 2 prunes,
    walnuts and ground flaxseeds
Green tea

### Lunch

Lamb's lettuce
Grilled steak
**Braised Carrots**

### Dinner

Grilled salmon with **Coriander Sauce**
Mixed green salad
Walnuts and goat's or sheep's cheese

# saturday

### Breakfast

**Super Vegetable Juice**
1 soft-boiled egg
1 slice Essene bread
Dandelion coffee

### Lunch

Radishes
Spelt bread sandwich with lettuce,
    tomatoes, tuna fish and **Mayonnaise**
**Pear Fruit Salad**

### Dinner

Mussels
Basmati rice
Dandelion leaf salad with walnuts and
    walnut oil
Fruit crumble

# sunday

### Breakfast

Papaya with lime juice
**Buckwheat Pancakes** – 3 with goat's
    cheese, 3 with maple syrup
Green tea

### Lunch

Lettuce salad
**Roast Chicken with Tarragon**
**Braised Fennel**
**Wild Rice**
**Quick Mango Sherbet**
Red wine

### Dinner

**Black Turtle Bean Soup with Parsley
    Sauce**
Spelt bread
1 fresh pear

# summer blood type o

## monday

### Breakfast

Peaches, raspberries and mango soya
    milkshake with 2 tablespoons
    ground flaxseeds

### Lunch

Tomatoes with basil and mozzarella
Grilled (broiled) sardines
**Spinach and Walnut Oil Salad**

### Dinner

Omelette with fresh herbs
**Broccoli with Ginger and Garlic**
Strawberries and peach fruit salad

## tuesday

### Breakfast

Apricots
Rye crackers with goat's cheese
Dandelion coffee

### Lunch

Grated beetroot (beet) salad
Grilled (broiled) steak
**Green Peas with Green Onions**
Raspberries

### Dinner

Steamed fish with lemon
Ratatouille
Basmati rice

## wednesday

### Breakfast

Nectarine
Scrambled egg
Spelt toast
Green tea

### Lunch

**Courgette Flower Fritters**
Lightly grilled (broiled) salmon with
    **Coriander Sauce**
**Spinach in Clarified Butter**

### Dinner

Rocket (arugula) salad with walnut oil
Grilled (broiled) duck leg
**Aubergine with Garlic and Thyme**
Blackcurrants

## thursday

### Breakfast

Blueberries
Essene bread with tahini
Goat's yogurt
Slippery elm tea

### Lunch

**Steak Tartare**
Tomato, fennel and green salad
Strawberries

### Dinner

**Grilled Marinated Tuna**
Grilled (broiled) tomatoes
Green salad
Fresh figs

# friday

**Breakfast**

Strawberries, nectarine and banana
  soya milkshake
Rye crackers
Mint tea

**Lunch**

Green salad
**Roast Chicken with Tarragon**
**Courgette Purée**

**Dinner**

**Marinated Grilled Peppers**
**Quinoa Tabbouleh**
Goat's cheese

# saturday

**Breakfast**

**Super Vegetable Juice**
Boiled egg
Toasted rye bread with butter
**Green Tea with Ginger**

**Lunch**

**Fish, Rice, Spinach and Onion Salad**
**Dark Plum Pie**

**Dinner**

**Salmon, Lime and Dill  Tartare**
Mixed green salad
Spelt bread
**Raspberry Sherbet**

# sunday

**Breakfast**

**Sourdough Pancakes** with blueberries
**Dandelion Coffee with Cardamom**

**Lunch**

**Green Bean Salad with Basil**
**Salmon Mousse**
**Curried Tomato Salad**
**Summer Red Fruit**
Wine

**Dinner**

Lamb chops
**Stuffed Courgettes**
Redcurrants and blackcurrants

# autumn blood type o

## monday

**Breakfast**

Grapes
Banana and date soya milkshake
**Green Tea with Ginger**

**Lunch**

Fennel Salad
Grilled (broiled) wild salmon
**Courgette Purée** with basil

**Dinner**

Rocket (arugula) salad with walnuts
    and walnut oil
Mushroom omelette
Fresh figs

## tuesday

**Breakfast**

1 slice pineapple
Essene bread and **Goat's Cheese
    Spread with Tarragon and Shallots**
Dandelion coffee and soya milk

**Lunch**

Grilled veal chops
Grilled (broiled) tomatoes
Green salad

**Dinner**

Steamed fillet of fish
**Spinach with Currants and Pine Nuts**
Apple sauce with ginger and
    cardamom

## wednesday

**Breakfast**

Grapes
Scrambled egg
Rye bread, toasted with butter
Mint tea

**Lunch**

Green salad
Grilled (broiled) steak
**Broccoli with Garlic and Ginger**

**Dinner**

**Chinese Chicken Broth**
**Tofu Salad**
**Dark Plum Pie**

## thursday

**Breakfast**

Soya milk mango shake with mixed
    flaxseeds and pumpkin seeds
Dandelion coffee

**Lunch**

**Raw Beetroot Salad**
**Monkfish en Papillote**
Basmati rice

**Dinner**

**Miso Soup**
**Chicken with Preserved Lemons**
**Braised Fennel**
Grapes

# friday

## Breakfast

1 pear
Essene bread
Mozzarella
**Green Tea with Ginger**

## Lunch

**Curried Tomato Salad**
Grilled (broiled) lamb chop
Green beans

## Dinner

**Fresh Bean and Onion Soup**
Endive salad with walnuts and walnut
    oil
Baked apples with raisins and ginger

# saturday

## Breakfast

**Super Vegetable Juice**
Toasted spelt bread
Boiled egg
Mint tea

## Lunch

Watercress salad
**Roast Venison**
**Braised Carrots with Fennel and
    Onions**
Raspberries

## Dinner

**Borsch**
Rye bread
**Plum Crumble**

# sunday

## Breakfast

**Sourdough Buckwheat Pancakes** and
    scalloped apples with spices
Sheep's yogurt
Vervain and mint tea

## Lunch

**Beetroot Salad with Walnuts and
    Roquefort**
**Wild Duck**
**Wild Rice**
**Celeriac and Parsley Purée**
**Autumn Apple Pie**
Red wine

## Dinner

**Black Turtle Bean Soup with
    Coriander Sauce**
Lamb's lettuce with hard-boiled egg
1 pear

# winter blood type o

## monday

### Breakfast

Oatmeal with raisins and soya milk
Mint tea

### Lunch

Grated celeriac with **Mayonnaise**
Steak
Steamed cabbage

### Dinner

**Fresh Bean and Onion Soup**
Scalloped apples with raisins and
    spices

## tuesday

### Breakfast

1 slice pineapple
Scrambled egg
1 slice spelt bread
Green tea

### Lunch

Lamb's lettuce
**Our Osso Buco**
**Braised Fennel**

### Dinner

Salad of winter greens
**Goat's Cheese Crêpes** with **Parsley
    Sauce**

## wednesday

### Breakfast

½ grapefruit
Essene bread with mozzarella cheese
**Green Tea with Ginger**

### Lunch

**Raw Beetroot Salad**
Lamb's kidneys
Basmati rice

### Dinner

Lamb's lettuce
**Guinea Fowl with Sage**
**Wild Rice**

## thursday

### Breakfast

½ mango
1 boiled egg
Rye crackers
Vervain tea

### Lunch

Grated carrots
Grilled (broiled) sardines
**Courgette Purée**

### Dinner

**Chicken with Lemon, Sage and Garlic**
**Celeriac and Parsley Purée**

# friday

### Breakfast

Miso Drink

Soya yogurt with chopped banana and
figs, pumpkin seeds and ground
flaxseeds

### Lunch

Grilled (broiled) lamb chops
Braised endives
1 slice **Three Ginger Cake**

### Dinner

6 oysters with rye bread
Steamed halibut or swordfish
**Braised Carrots with Fennel and
Onions**
Apple sauce
**Cinnamon Stars**

# saturday

### Breakfast

**Super Vegetable Juice**
Scrambled egg
Spelt bread
Mint tea

### Lunch

**Winter Salad with Prunes and Apricots**
**Monkfish en Papillote**
Basmati rice
**Poached Pears in Citrus Juice and
Grand Marnier**

### Dinner

**Winter White Bean Soup**
**Chocolate Delight**

# sunday

### Breakfast

**Sourdough Buckwheat Pancakes** with
sheep's yogurt and apple sauce

### Lunch

Green salad
**Guinea Fowl with Sage**
**Roasted Winter Vegetables**
**Apple Walnut Maple Syrup Pie**
Red wine

### Dinner

**Miso Soup**
**Onion Pancakes**
Endive salad
Goat's cheese

# spring blood type a

## monday

### Breakfast

½ grapefruit
1 slice Essene bread with goat's cheese
Green tea

### Lunch

**Broccoli Velouté**
**Tofu Salad**
Dates, figs and walnuts

### Dinner

Steamed fish fillet with **Parsley Sauce**
Spinach with raisins and hazelnuts
Pear

## tuesday

### Breakfast

1 slice pineapple
Soya yogurt with walnuts, flaxseeds,
    pumpkin and sunflower seeds
Rose hip tea

### Lunch

**Raw Beetroot Salad**
Omelette with chopped chervil
**Broccoli with Ginger and Garlic**

### Dinner

**Miso Soup**
Soba noodles
Green salad
Prunes

## wednesday

### Breakfast

1 apple
2 slices toasted spelt bread with peanut
    butter
**Green Tea with Ginger**

### Lunch

**Fennel Salad**
**Grilled Tuna** with **Ginger and Tamari
    Sauce**
Green beans
Sheep's yogurt

### Dinner

Fresh asparagus
**Guinea Fowl with Sage**
**Courgette Purée**
Polenta
Pineapple

## thursday

### Breakfast

1 kiwi fruit
Scrambled egg with 1 slice toasted rye
    bread
Coffee with soya milk

### Lunch

Avocado salad
**Marinated Tempeh**
Brown rice

### Dinner

Spinach salad
**Goat's Cheese Dumplings**
Strawberries

# friday

## Breakfast

1 bowl of cherries

1 soya yogurt with sunflower seeds, two
tablespoons of ground flaxseeds and
maple syrup

Ginger tea

## Lunch

Lamb's lettuce salad

**Marinated Tofu Brochettes**

Basmati rice

## Dinner

Grilled (broiled) salmon with **Fresh
Coriander Sauce**

Mixed green salad

Walnuts and goat's or sheep's cheese

# saturday

## Breakfast

**Super Vegetable Juice**

1 boiled egg

Rye crackers

Green tea

## Lunch

Radishes

Spelt bread sandwich with lettuce,
green onions, tuna and **Mayonnaise**

Pear salad

## Dinner

**Snails with Oregano and Shallots**

Dandelion salad with walnuts

Fruit crumble (see **Plum Crumble**)

# sunday

## Breakfast

1 slice pineapple

**Sourdough Buckwheat Pancakes** –
3 goat's cheese, 3 maple syrup

Coffee with goat's milk

## Lunch

Green lettuce salad

**Roast Chicken with Tarragon**

**Braised Fennel**

**Wild Rice**

**Raspberry Sherbet**

Red wine

## Dinner

**Black Turtle Bean Soup** with **Parsley
Sauce**

Apple sauce with goat's yogurt

## monday

### Breakfast

Peach, strawberry, soya milkshake with
    2 tablespoons ground flaxseeds
Green tea

### Lunch

Grilled (broiled) sardines
**Spinach and Walnut Oil Salad**
Nectarine

### Dinner

Artichoke pasta with **Basil Sauce**
Rocket (arugula) salad
Blueberries

## tuesday

### Breakfast

Apricots
2 slices toasted rye bread
Goat's cheese
**Green Tea with Ginger**

### Lunch

Green salad
**Chicken with Preserved Lemons**
Basmati rice
**Chocolate Delight**

### Dinner

**Chinese Chicken Broth**
**Tofu Salad**
Strawberries and peach fruit salad

## wednesday

### Breakfast

Raspberries
Scrambled egg
Toasted spelt bread
Green tea

### Lunch

**Courgette Flower Fritters**
Steamed salmon with **Soya Yogurt Dill
    Sauce**
**Spinach in Clarified Butter**

### Dinner

Wild mushroom omelette
Watercress salad with hazelnut oil
Goat's cheese

## thursday

### Breakfast

Blueberries
Goat's yogurt
Essene bread with tahini
Ginseng tea

### Lunch

**Chilled Avocado Soup**
**Marinated Tempeh**
Green beans

### Dinner

**Quinoa Tabbouleh** (without tomatoes)
**Grilled Tuna**
Steamed courgette (zucchini) with
    garlic and olive oil
Blackcurrants

# friday

## Breakfast

Blackberries
Soya yogurt
Rye crackers with peanut butter

## Lunch

**Lentil Salad**
**Roast Chicken with Tarragon**
**Green Peas with Green Onions**

## Dinner

Steamed tofu with **Ginger and Tamari Sauce**
Basmati rice
Fresh figs

# saturday

## Breakfast

**Super Vegetable Juice**
Soya yogurt with pumpkin seeds
**Green Tea with Ginger**

## Lunch

**Fish, Rice, Spinach and Onion Salad**
**Dark Plum Pie**

## Dinner

**Salmon, Lime and Dill Tartare**
Mixed green salad
Toasted spelt bread
**Raspberry Sherbet**

# sunday

## Breakfast

**Sourdough Pancakes** with blueberries
Yogurt
Coffee

## Lunch

**Salmon Mousse**
**Cucumber Raita with Grilled Cumin Seeds**
**Green Bean Salad with Basil**
**Summer Red Fruit**
Red wine

## Dinner

**Stuffed Courgettes**
Mixed green salad
Redcurrants and blackcurrants

## monday

### Breakfast

Soya milk, pear and prune shake with 2
tablespoons of ground flaxseeds
**Green Tea with Ginger**

### Lunch

**Fennel Salad**
Grilled (broiled) wild salmon
**Courgette Purée** with basil
Rice

### Dinner

Mushroom omelette
Rocket (arugula) salad with walnuts
and walnut oil
Fresh figs

## tuesday

### Breakfast

Grapes
Essene bread and **Goat's Cheese with
Tarragon and Shallots**

### Lunch

**Lentil Salad with Fennel, Parsley and
Coriander**
Soya yogurt

### Dinner

Steamed fish
Spinach with raisins and hazelnuts
Apple sauce with ginger and
cardamom

## wednesday

### Breakfast

1 slice pineapple
1 scrambled egg
Rye crackers
Green tea

### Lunch

Green salad
**Grilled Tuna** with **Basil Sauce**
**Broccoli with Garlic and Ginger**
Quinoa

### Dinner

**Chinese Chicken Broth**
**Tofu Salad**
**Dark Plum Pie**

## thursday

### Breakfast

Blackberries with yogurt
Spelt bread with tahini
Rose hip tea

### Lunch

**Raw Beetroot Salad**
**Monkfish en Papillote**
**Braised Fennel**
Yogurt with apple sauce

### Dinner

**Miso Soup**
**Chicken with Preserved Lemons**
Basmati rice
Grapes

# friday

## Breakfast

1 pear
Essene bread with mozzarella cheese
**Green Tea with Ginger**

## Lunch

Ostrich roast
Steamed turnips, carrots and
   courgettes (zucchini) with **Aïoli**

## Dinner

**Fresh Bean and Onion Soup**
Endive salad with walnuts and walnut
   oil
Baked apples with raisins and ginger

# saturday

## Breakfast

**Super Vegetable Juice**
1 boiled egg
Toasted rye bread with **Clarified Butter**
Vervain tea

## Lunch

Watercress salad
**Marinated Tofu Brochettes with
   Thyme and Oregano**
**Braised Carrots with Fennel and
   Onions**
Raspberries with sour cream

## Dinner

**Borsch** (without meat)
Rye bread
Goat's cheese
**Plum Crumble**

# sunday

## Breakfast

**Sourdough Buckwheat Pancakes** and
   apple sauce with ginger and
   cardamom
Sheep's yogurt
Coffee

## Lunch

**Beetroot Salad with Walnuts and
   Roquefort**
**Roast Chicken with Tarragon**
**Wild Rice**
**Celeriac and Parsley Purée**
**Autumn Apple Pie**
Red wine

## Dinner

**Black Turtle Bean Soup with Fresh
   Coriander Sauce**
Lamb's lettuce with 1 hard-boiled egg
Baked apples with raisins and ginger

# winter blood type a

## monday

### Breakfast

Grapefruit juice
Buckwheat porridge with pumpkin
   seeds
Green tea

### Lunch

**Miso Soup**
**Tofu Salad**

### Dinner

**Fresh Bean and Onion Soup**
Baked apple with raisins and spices

## tuesday

### Breakfast

Soya milkshake with molasses, dried
   apricots and pear
Rye crackers
Rose hip tea

### Lunch

Beetroot salad with walnuts and goat's
   cheese
Omelette

### Dinner

Grilled (broiled) turkey
Steamed leek, carrot, parsnip and
   turnip with **Aïoli**
Dried figs and apricots

## wednesday

### Breakfast

1 kiwi
Oatmeal porridge with sesame seeds
Coffee with soya milk

### Lunch

Grated raw carrots
Grilled (broiled) sardines
**Courgette Purée**

### Dinner

**Chinese Chicken Broth**
**Pan-fried Tempeh**
Lamb's lettuce
**Almond and Raisin Biscuits (Cookies)**

## thursday

### Breakfast

1 slice pineapple
Scrambled egg
**Green Tea with Ginger**

### Lunch

Grated celeriac with **Mayonnaise**
**Chicken with Lemon, Sage and Garlic**
**Braised Fennel**

### Dinner

Salad of winter greens
**Goat's Cheese Crêpes with Green
   Sauce**
**Pear Fruit Salad**

# friday

### Breakfast

1 apple
**Miso Drink**
Essene bread with peanut butter

### Lunch

**Broccoli Velouté**
**Lentil Salad with Fennel and Herbs**
Stewed prunes

### Dinner

**Baked Fish with Shallots and Ginger**
**Braised Carrots with Fennel and
    Onions**
Apple sauce
**Cinnamon Stars**

# saturday

### Breakfast

**Super Vegetable Juice**
1 boiled egg
Rye bread
Ginseng tea

### Lunch

**Winter Salad with Prunes and Apricots**
**Monkfish** with **Coriander Sauce**
Basmati rice
**Poached Pears in Citrus Juice and
    Grand Marnier**

### Dinner

**Winter White Bean Soup**
Escarole salad
**Chocolate Delight**

# sunday

### Breakfast

**Sourdough Buckwheat Pancakes** with
    goat's yogurt and apple sauce
Coffee with soya milk

### Lunch

Mixed winter green salad
**Guinea Fowl with Sage**
**Roasted Winter Vegetables**
**Apple, Walnut and Maple Syrup Pie**
Red wine

### Dinner

**Miso Soup**
**Onion Pancakes**
Endive salad
Goat's cheese with rye crackers

## monday

### Breakfast

½ grapefruit
Essene bread with cheese of your
    choice
**Green Tea with Ginger**

### Lunch

**Broccoli Velouté**
Steak
Green salad
Dates, figs and walnuts
Coffee

### Dinner

Steamed fish with **Parsley Sauce**
**Spinach with raisins and grilled
    (broiled) almonds**
Fresh pear

## tuesday

### Breakfast

1 slice pineapple
Yogurt with black walnuts, chopped
    banana and ground flaxseeds
Green tea

### Lunch

**Raw Beetroot Salad**
Grilled (broiled) lamb chops
**Steamed Broccoli with Ginger and
    Garlic**

### Dinner

**Rabbit with Provençale Herbs**
Baked sweet potato
Green salad

## wednesday

### Breakfast

1 papaya with lime juice
1 scrambled egg
1 slice spelt bread
Dandelion coffee with milk

### Lunch

**Fennel Salad**
**Grilled Tuna** with **Ginger and Tamari
    Sauce**
**Cucumber Raita with Grilled Cumin
    Seeds**
Basmati rice

### Dinner

Fresh asparagus
**Braised Lamb with Onions and Lemon**
1 slice pineapple

## thursday

### Breakfast

1 kiwi fruit
Oatmeal porridge with milk and raisins
Coffee

### Lunch

Endive, apple and walnut salad
Calves' liver
Green beans

### Dinner

Spinach salad
**Goat's Cheese Dumplings**
Strawberries and sour cream

# friday

## Breakfast

1 bowl cherries
Essene bread with butter
Yogurt
**Green Tea with Ginger**

## Lunch

Lamb's lettuce
Grilled (broiled) mackerel
Steamed potato

## Dinner

Mixed green salad
Grilled (broiled) lamb chops
Walnuts and cheese on bread
Apple sauce

# saturday

## Breakfast

**Super Vegetable Juice**
1 soft-boiled egg
Spelt toast and mozzarella
Green tea

## Lunch

**Pear, Walnut and Parmesan Salad**
**Rabbit with Preserved Lemons**
Braised carrots

## Dinner

Grilled (broiled) salmon with **Fresh
    Coriander Sauce**
Basmati rice
Dandelion salad with walnut oil
Fruit crumble (see **Plum Crumble**)

# sunday

## Breakfast

1 orange
**Sourdough Spelt Pancakes** with goat's
    cheese or maple syrup
Coffee

## Lunch

Spring lettuce salad
**Marinated Shoulder of Lamb**
**Braised Fennel**
Basmati rice
**Quick Mango Sherbet**
Red wine

## Dinner

**Fresh Bean and Onion Soup**
**Pear Fruit Salad**

# summer blood type b

## monday

**Breakfast**

Peach and strawberry soya milkshake
with 2 tablespoons of ground
flaxseeds
Green tea

**Lunch**

**Spinach and Walnut Oil Salad**
Lamb chops
Green beans
Nectarine

**Dinner**

Wild mushroom omelette
Watercress salad
Cheese

## tuesday

**Breakfast**

Apricots
Spelt bread and **Goat's Cheese with
Tarragon and Shallots**
Raspberry leaf tea

**Lunch**

Cucumber salad
**Rabbit with Preserved Lemons**
**Saffron Potatoes**

**Dinner**

**Grilled Tuna** with **Ginger and Tamari
Sauce**
Basmati rice
Strawberries and cream

## wednesday

**Breakfast**

Raspberries
Scrambled egg
Essene bread
**Green Tea with Ginger**

**Lunch**

**Courgette Flower Fritters**
**Monkfish en Papillote** with **Fresh
Coriander Sauce**
**Spinach in Clarified Butter**

**Dinner**

**Steak Tartare**
Mixed green salad
Spelt bread
Goat's yogurt with blackstrap molasses

## thursday

**Breakfast**

Puffed rice with blueberries and
banana
Kefir
Rose hip tea

**Lunch**

Grilled (broiled) steak
**Green Bean Salad with Basil**
**Chocolate Delight**

**Dinner**

Pasta with **Parsley Sauce**
Rocket (arugula) salad
Goat's cheese
Summer fruit salad

# friday

## Breakfast

Raspberries
Toasted spelt bread
Cheese
Mint tea

## Lunch

**Fish, Rice, Spinach and Onion Salad**
**Dark Plum Pie**

## Dinner

Grilled (broiled) turkey breast with
    **Fresh Coriander Sauce**
**Courgette Purée**
Peaches and ricotta cheese

# saturday

## Breakfast

**Super Vegetable Juice**
Oatcakes
Feta cheese
Black tea

## Lunch

Grilled (broiled) lamb chops
**Aubergine with Garlic and Thyme**
**Oven Fries**

## Dinner

**Salmon, Lime and Dill Tartare**
Mixed green salad
**Raspberry Sherbet**

# sunday

## Breakfast

**Sourdough Pancakes** with blueberries
Sheep's yogurt
Coffee

## Lunch

**Marinated Grilled Peppers**
**Salmon Mousse**
**Cucumber Raita with Grilled Cumin
    Seeds**
Summer Red Fruit
Wine

## Dinner

Veal chops
**Vegetables with Rosemary**
Mixed green salad
Spelt bread with cheese

## monday

**Breakfast**

Grapes
Oatmeal porridge
Milk
**Dandelion Coffee with Cardamom**

**Lunch**

Coleslaw
Grilled (broiled) sardines
Mashed potatoes

**Dinner**

Autumn mushroom omelette
Rocket (arugula) salad with walnuts
and walnut oil
Pear

## tuesday

**Breakfast**

Figs
Essene bread with mozzarella
Raspberry leaf tea

**Lunch**

Grated carrots
Grilled (broiled) lamb chops
Green beans
Goat's yogurt

**Dinner**

**Goat's Cheese Dumplings**
**Spinach and Walnut Oil Salad**
Grapes

## wednesday

**Breakfast**

Orange juice
Boiled egg
Spelt bread, toasted
Peppermint tea

**Lunch**

**Fennel Salad**
**Rabbit with Preserved Lemons**
Basmati rice

**Dinner**

Grilled (broiled) mackerel
**Celeriac and Parsley Purée**
**Plum Crumble**

## thursday

**Breakfast**

Plums
Brown rice with olive oil and tamari
Rose hip tea

**Lunch**

**Beetroot Salad with Walnuts and
Roquefort**
Calves' liver
**Braised Carrots with Fennel and
Onions**

**Dinner**

**Monkfish en Papillote**
Tagliatelle with **Parsley Sauce**
Baked apples

# friday

### Breakfast

Pears with walnuts
Goat's yogurt with 2 tablespoons
  ground flaxseeds
Licorice tea

### Lunch

Grilled (broiled) turkey
**Braised Fennel**
**Autumn Apple Pie**

### Dinner

Belgian endive, apple and walnut salad
Steak
**Oven Fries**

# saturday

### Breakfast

**Super Vegetable Juice**
Oatcakes
Goat's cheese spread
**Green Tea with Ginger**

### Lunch

Steamed fish
Steamed potatoes with **Aïoli**
Escarole salad
Raspberries and cream

### Dinner

**Rabbit with Provençale Herbs**
**Braised Fennel Bulbs**
**Poached Pears in Citrus Fruit and
  Grand Marnier**

# sunday

### Breakfast

**Sourdough Spelt Pancakes** with apple
  sauce
Sheep's yogurt
Coffee

### Lunch

**Pear, Walnut and Parmesan Salad**
**Roast Venison**
**Celeriac and Parsley Purée**
Cranberry sauce
**Dark Plum Pie**

### Dinner

**Winter White Bean Soup**
Bread and cheese

# winter blood type b

## monday

### Breakfast

½ grapefruit
Oatmeal porridge with raisins and
   cinnamon
Milk
Green tea

### Lunch

Grated beetroots (beets)
Hamburger steak with **Parsley Sauce**
Mashed potatoes with garlic
Yogurt

### Dinner

Calves' liver
**Roasted Winter Vegetables**
**Quick Mango Sherbet**
**Almond and Raisin Biscuits (Cookies)**

## tuesday

### Breakfast

Stewed prunes
Essene bread with mozzarella
Ginger tea

### Lunch

Grilled (broiled) fish
**Broccoli with Garlic and Ginger**
Apple sauce

### Dinner

Vegetable soup
Salad with hard-boiled egg
Cheese
Grapes

## wednesday

### Breakfast

Fresh pineapple
Spelt bread and **Goat's Cheese with
   Tarragon and Shallots**
Raspberry leaf tea

### Lunch

Lamb's lettuce
**Braised Lamb with Onions and Lemons**
**Saffron Potatoes**

### Dinner

Grated celeriac with **Mayonnaise**
Grilled (broiled) turkey
**Vegetables in Olive Oil**
Baked apple

## thursday

### Breakfast

Papaya with lime juice
Scrambled egg
Oatcakes
**Dandelion Coffee with Cardamom**

### Lunch

**Broccoli Velouté**
**Our Osso Buco**
Basmati rice
Dried figs and walnuts

### Dinner

Romaine salad with feta
Steamed fish with **Parsley Sauce**
**Braised Fennel**
**Poached Pears in Citrus Fruit and
   Grand Marnier**

# friday

### Breakfast

2 kiwi fruit
Spelt bread, toasted
Sheep's yogurt with blackstrap
 molasses
Rose hip tea

### Lunch

**Winter Salad with Walnuts, Prunes
 and Dried Apricots**
Grilled (broiled) salmon
**Spinach in Clarified Butter**

### Dinner

Chicory salad with apple
**Rabbit with Preserved Lemons**
**Wild Rice**
Dates

# saturday

### Breakfast

**Super Vegetable Juice**
Oatmeal porridge with dried figs and
 apricots
**Green Tea with Ginger**

### Lunch

**Borsch**
Spelt bread with cheese

### Dinner

Roasted pheasant
**Celeriac and Parsley Purée**
Belgian endive salad
Fresh pineapple
Slice of **Christmas Fruit Cake**

# sunday

### Breakfast

**Sourdough Spelt Pancakes**
**Goat's Cheese with Tarragon and
 Shallots**
Coffee

### Lunch

Lamb's lettuce
**Braised Beef**
**Apple, Walnut and Maple Syrup Pie**

### Dinner

**Fresh Bean and Onion Soup**
**Pear Fruit Salad**
**Cinnamon Stars**

## spring blood type ab

### monday

**Breakfast**

½ grapefruit
1 slice Essene bread
Goat's cheese
Green tea

**Lunch**

**Broccoli Velouté**
**Tofu Salad**
Dates, figs and walnuts

**Dinner**

Grilled (broiled) sardines
Spinach with raisins and hazelnuts
Pear

### tuesday

**Breakfast**

1 slice pineapple
Yogurt with walnuts and chopped
    almonds
Rose hip tea

**Lunch**

**Raw Beetroot Salad**
Omelette with chopped chervil
**Broccoli with Garlic and Ginger**

**Dinner**

**Miso Soup**
Baked sweet potato
Green salad
Kiwi fruit salad

### wednesday

**Breakfast**

1 apple
2 slices wheat bread with peanut butter
**Green Tea with Ginger**

**Lunch**

**Cucumber Raita with Cumin**
**Grilled Tuna with Ginger and Tamari**
    **Sauce**
Green beans

**Dinner**

Fresh asparagus
**Rabbit with Preserved Lemons**
**Courgette Purée**
1 slice pineapple

### thursday

**Breakfast**

1 kiwi fruit
Scrambled egg
Toasted rye bread
Coffee with soya milk

**Lunch**

**Fennel Salad**
**Marinated Tempeh**
Brown rice

**Dinner**

Spinach salad
**Goat's Cheese Dumplings**
Strawberries and sour cream

# friday

## Breakfast

Cherries
Goat's yogurt with maple syrup
Whole-grain rye crackers
**Green Tea with Ginger**

## Lunch

Dandelion salad
**Marinated Tofu Brochettes**
Basmati rice

## Dinner

Grilled (broiled) salmon with **Fresh
    Coriander Sauce**
Mixed green salad
Walnuts and cheddar cheese

# saturday

## Breakfast

**Super Vegetable Juice**
Boiled egg
Essene bread
Green tea

## Lunch

Spelt bread sandwich with lettuce,
    green onions, tuna and **Mayonnaise**
**Pear Fruit Salad**

## Dinner

Snails with oregano and shallots
Endive salad with walnut oil
Fruit crumble (see **Plum Crumble**)

# sunday

## Breakfast

Cranberry juice or 1 slice pineapple
**Spelt Pancakes** with goat's cheese or
    maple syrup
Coffee with goat's milk

## Lunch

Spring lettuce salad
**Marinated Shoulder of Lamb**
**Braised Fennel**
**Wild Rice**
**Raspberry Sherbet**
Red wine

## Dinner

**Fresh Bean and Onion soup**
Apple sauce with sour cream

## monday

### Breakfast

Peach strawberry soya milkshake with
2 tablespoons of ground flaxseeds

### Lunch

**Spinach Salad in Walnut Oil**
Grilled (broiled) lamb chops
Grilled (broiled) tomatoes
Nectarine

### Dinner

Green salad
**Monkfish en Papillote** with **Fresh
Coriander Sauce**
**Saffron Potatoes**
Raspberries with low fat sour cream

## tuesday

### Breakfast

Apricots
Toasted rye bread and **Goat's Cheese
with Tarragon and Shallots**
Green tea

### Lunch

**Broccoli Velouté**, chilled
**Tofu Salad**
Yogurt

### Dinner

Tomato salad
Pasta with **Basil Sauce**
Goat's cheese

## wednesday

### Breakfast

Strawberries
Scrambled egg
Essene bread with mozzarella cheese
Ginger tea

### Lunch

**Green Bean Salad with Basil**
**Grilled Tuna** with **Fresh Coriander
Sauce**
Blueberries

### Dinner

**Baked Fish with Shallots and Ginger**
**Wild Rice**
Green salad with rocket (arugula)
Yogurt

## thursday

### Breakfast

Peach
Oatcakes with feta cheese
Green tea

### Lunch

Green salad
Snails with oregano and shallots
Basmati rice
Watermelon

### Dinner

Cucumber salad
Grilled (broiled) turkey breast with
**Fresh Coriander Sauce**
**Oven Fries**
Summer fruit salad

# friday

## Breakfast

Cottage cheese with nectarine and
    raspberries
Ryo crackers
Rose hip tea

## Lunch

**Lentil Salad with Fennel and Herbs**
Green salad with hard-boiled egg
Sheep's milk yogurt

## Dinner

**Rabbit with Preserved Lemons**
**Courgette Purée**
Basmati rice
**Spicy Peaches in Red Wine**

# saturday

## Breakfast

**Super Vegetable Juice**
Boiled egg
Spelt toast
Kefir
**Green Tea with Ginger**

## Lunch

**Marinated Tempeh**
**Aubergine with Garlic and Thyme**
Goat's cheese

## Dinner

**Salmon, Lime and Dill Tartare**
Mixed green salad
**Raspberry Sherbet**

# sunday

## Breakfast

**Sourdough Pancakes** with blueberries
Goat's yogurt

## Lunch

**Salmon Mousse**
**Cucumber Raita with Cumin Seeds**
**Curried Tomato Salad**
**Summer Red Fruit**

## Dinner

Grilled (broiled) lamb chops
**Stuffed Courgette**
Watermelon

## monday

**Breakfast**

Grapes
Oatmeal porridge with raisins and
    cinnamon
Semi-skimmed (2% fat) milk
**Dandelion Coffee with Cardamom**

**Lunch**

Tomato salad
Grilled (broiled) sardines
Mashed potatoes

**Dinner**

Autumn mushroom omelette
Rocket (arugula) salad with walnuts
    and walnut oil
Pear

## tuesday

**Breakfast**

Fresh figs
Essene bread with mozzarella
Green tea

**Lunch**

Watercress salad
Calves' liver
**Braised Carrots**
Yogurt

**Dinner**

**Goat's Cheese Dumplings**
**Spinach Salad in Walnut Oil**
Grapes

## wednesday

**Breakfast**

½ grapefruit
Scrambled egg on rye toast
Rose hip tea

**Lunch**

**Fennel Salad**
Lentils
Basmati rice
Cheese

**Dinner**

Grilled (broiled) mackerel
**Celeriac and Parsley Purée**
**Plum Crumble**

## thursday

**Breakfast**

Plums
Rye crackers
**Goat's Cheese with Tarragon and
    Shallots**
**Green Tea with Ginger**

**Lunch**

Grated carrots
Grilled (broiled) lamb chops
Green beans
Pear

**Dinner**

**Monkfish en Papillote**
Steamed cauliflower with **Parsley
    Sauce**
Baked apples with spices and raisins

# friday

### Breakfast

Grapes
Cottage cheese with cinnamon,
    walnuts and dried figs
Licorice tea

### Lunch

Grilled (broiled) turkey
**Braised Carrots with Fennel and
    Onion**
**Autumn Apple Pie**

### Dinner

Chicory, apple and walnut salad
Mussels
**Oven Fries**

# saturday

### Breakfast

**Super Vegetable Juice**
Toasted spelt bread with sheep's cheese
    and tomato
Dandelion coffee

### Lunch

Escarole salad
Steamed fish
Steamed potato with **Aïoli**
Raspberries with sour cream

### Dinner

**Rabbit with Provençale Herbs**
**Braised Fennel Bulbs**
**Poached Pears in Citrus Juice and
    Grand Marnier**

# sunday

### Breakfast

**Sourdough Spelt Pancakes**
Apple sauce
Sheep's yogurt
Green tea

### Lunch

**Pear, Walnut and Parmesan Salad**
**Roast Venison**
**Celeriac and Parsley Purée**
**Dark Plum Pie**

### Dinner

**Winter White Bean Soup**
Bread and cheese

## monday

### Breakfast

½ grapefruit
Oatmeal porridge with raisins and
   cinnamon
Semi-skimmed (2% fat) milk
Green tea

### Lunch

**Raw Beetroot Salad**
Grilled (broiled) mackerel with
   provençale herbs
Mashed potatoes
Goat's yogurt

### Dinner

Calves' liver
**Roasted Winter Vegetables**
Pear
**Almond and Raisin Biscuits (Cookies)**

## tuesday

### Breakfast

Stewed prunes
Toasted rye bread
**Goat's Cheese with Tarragon and
   Shallots**
**Green Tea with Ginger**

### Lunch

Grilled (broiled) turkey
**Broccoli with Ginger and Garlic**
Apple sauce

### Dinner

Vegetable soup
**Baked Fish with Shallots and Ginger**
**Braised Fennel**
Grapes

## wednesday

### Breakfast

Slice fresh pineapple
Spelt bread with peanut butter and honey
Soya yogurt
Dandelion coffee

### Lunch

**Chinese Turkey Broth**
**Marinated Tofu Brochettes with
   Thyme and Oregano**
Basmati rice
**Vegetables in Olive Oil**

### Dinner

Lamb's lettuce
**Rabbit with Preserved Lemons**
**Wild Rice**
Baked apple

## thursday

### Breakfast

Papaya with lime juice
Scrambled egg
Rye crackers
Strawberry leaf tea

### Lunch

**Fennel Salad**
Lentils
**Spinach with Currants and Pine Nuts**
Cheese

### Dinner

**Broccoli Velouté**
Grilled (broiled) lamb chop
Braised chicory
**Poached Pears in Citrus Juice and
    Grand Marnier**
**Hazelnut Leckerli**

## friday

### Breakfast

2 kiwi fruit
Toasted spelt bread with honey
Sheep's yogurt
Rose hip tea

### Lunch

**Winter Salad with Prunes and Apricots**
Steamed fish with **Parsley Sauce**
Steamed potatoes

### Dinner

Omelette
**Braised Carrots with Fennel and
    Onions**
Apple sauce

## saturday

### Breakfast

**Super Vegetable Juice**
Oatcakes with goat's cheese
**Dandelion Coffee with Cardamom**

### Lunch

Roast pheasant
**Celeriac Purée with Parsley**
Fresh pineapple
Slice of **Christmas Fruit Cake**

### Dinner

**Borsch** (without meat)
Goat's cheese
Baked apples with raisins and ginger

## sunday

### Breakfast

**Sourdough Spelt Pancakes**
**Goat's Cheese with Tarragon and
    Shallots**
Green tea

### Lunch

Lamb's lettuce
**Braised Lamb with Onions and
    Lemons**
**Saffron Potatoes in Lemon Juice**
Apple, Walnut and Maple Syrup Pie

### Dinner

**Fresh Bean and Onion Soup**
**Pear Fruit Salad**
**Cinnamon Stars**

# seven individual days for all blood types

Here we have created seven days of menus that are suitable for all blood types. At first thought feeding several blood types may seem a hassle, but if you approach this obstacle with a creative mind you will enjoy the satisfaction of catering to the health of all those at your table.

It is important to stress, however, that these menus cannot be followed by all types on a regular basis as each blood type would miss out on a great many beneficial foods.

## day 1

### Breakfast

½ grapefruit
Scrambled egg
Essene bread
Green tea

### Lunch

**Gravlax** with toasted spelt bread
Mixed green salad
Grated carrots
Strawberries

### Dinner

**Broccoli Velouté**
Grilled Cod
**Braised Fennel Bulbs**
**Spicy Peaches in Red Wine**

## day 2

### Breakfast

1 slice pineapple
Spelt toast and **Goat's Cheese with Tarragon and Shallots**
Peppermint tea

### Lunch

Grilled (broiled) turkey
**Braised Carrots, Fennel and Onions**
Pear

### Dinner

**Raw Beetroot Salad**
**Monkfish en Papillote**
**Spinach in Clarified Butter**
Baked apples

## day 3

### Breakfast

1 apple
1 boiled egg
Essene bread
Dandelion coffee

### Lunch

**Fennel Salad**
**Grilled Tuna** with **Ginger and Tamari Sauce**
Basmati rice
Peach

### Dinner

Lamb's lettuce
**Onion Pancakes**
**Roasted Winter Vegetables**
Figs and walnuts

# day 4

## Breakfast

Cherries

Sheep's yogurt with molasses and
    walnuts

Rose hip tea

## Lunch

Turkey meat balls

**Celeriac Purée with Parsley**

Brown basmati rice

Grapes

## Dinner

**Fish, Rice, Spinach and Onion Salad**

**Plum Crumble**

# day 5

## Breakfast

Apple, pear and grapefruit fresh fruit
    salad

Scrambled egg

Green tea

## Lunch

**Baked Fish with Shallots and Ginger**

**Spinach in Clarified Butter**

Basmati rice

1 slice pineapple

## Dinner

**Chinese Turkey Broth**

Grilled (broiled) fresh sardines

**Vegetables with Rosemary**

# day 6

## Breakfast

**Super Vegetable Juice** – carrot, celery,
    beetroot, lemon and ginger

Essene bread with mozzarella

**Dandelion Coffee with Cardamom**

## Lunch

Green bean salad

Ostrich roast

**Courgette Purée**

Quinoa

## Dinner

**Salmon, Lime and Dill Tartare**

Mixed green salad

Spelt bread

**Raspberry Sherbet**

# day 7

## Breakfast

**Sourdough Spelt Pancakes** with
    sheep's yogurt and blueberries

**Green Tea with Ginger**

## Lunch

**Salmon Mousse**

**Quinoa Tabbouleh**

**Spinach and Walnut Oil Salad**

**Summer Red Fruit**

Wine

## Dinner

**Winter White Bean Soup**

Seasonal green salad

Baked apples with raisins and ginger

# recipe list

| **Soups** | **O** | **A** | **B** | **AB** |
|---|---|---|---|---|
| Borsch (if made with lamb) (page 50) | + | | + | + |
| Broccoli velouté (page 52) | + | + | + | + |
| Chilled avocado soup (page 53) | | + | + | |
| Chinese chicken or turkey broth (page 54) | + | + | + | + |
| Miso soup (page 55) | + | + | | + |
| Black turtle bean soup (page 58) | + | + | | |
| Winter white bean soup (page 59) | + | + | + | + |
| Fresh bean and onion soup (page 60) | + | + | + | + |

| **Salads** | **O** | **A** | **B** | **AB** |
|---|---|---|---|---|
| Beetroot salad with walnuts and roquefort (page 65) | + | + | + | + |
| Cucumber raita with grilled cumin seeds (page 66) | | + | + | + |
| Fennel salad (page 67) | + | + | + | + |
| Fish, rice, spinach and onion salad (using a common fish) (page 68) | + | + | + | + |
| Green bean salad with basil (page 69) | + | + | + | + |
| Lentil salad with fennel and herbs (page 70) | | + | | + |
| Marinated grilled peppers (page 71) | + | | + | |
| Pear, walnut and parmesan salad (using a hard sheep's cheese instead of Parmigiano Reggiano) (page 72) | + | + | + | + |
| Quinoa tabbouleh (page 73) | + | + | + | + |
| Raw beetroot salad (page 74) | + | + | + | + |
| Spinach salad in walnut oil (page 75) | + | + | + | + |
| Tofu salad (page 76) | + | + | | + |
| Curried tomato salad (page 77) | + | | | + |
| Winter salad with walnuts, prunes and apricots (page 78) | + | + | + | + |

| Vegetables | O | A | B | AB |
|---|---|---|---|---|
| Braised carrots (page 81) | + | + | + | + |
| Braised carrots, fennel and onions (page 82) | + | + | + | + |
| Braised fennel bulbs (page 83) | + | + | + | + |
| Broccoli with garlic and ginger (page 84) | + | + | + | + |
| Celeriac purée with parsley (page 85) | + | + | + | + |
| Aubergine with garlic and thyme (page 86) | + | | + | + |
| End-of-holiday vegetables (page 87) | + | + | + | + |
| Green peas and green onions (page 88) | + | + | + | + |
| Onion pancakes (page 89) | + | + | + | + |
| Oven fries (page 90) | | | + | + |
| Roasted winter vegetables (page 91) | + | + | + | + |
| Saffron potatoes in lemon juice (page 92) | | | + | + |
| Spinach in clarified butter (page 93) | + | + | + | + |
| Spinach with currants and pine nuts (page 94) | + | + | + | + |
| Stuffed courgette flowers (page 95) | + | + | + | + |
| Stuffed courgettes (page 96) | + | | | + |
| Vegetables in olive oil (page 97) | | + | + | + |
| Vegetables with rosemary (page 98) | + | + | + | + |
| Wild rice (page 99) | + | + | | + |
| Courgette flower fritters (page 100) | + | + | + | + |
| Courgette purée (page 100) | + | + | + | + |

| Goat's Cheese | O | A | B | AB |
|---|---|---|---|---|
| Crêpes with goat's cheese and green sauce (page 102) | + | + | + | + |
| Goat's cheese dumplings (page 103) | + | + | + | + |
| Goat's cheese with tarragon and shallots (page 104) | + | + | + | + |

| Snails | O | A | B | AB |
|---|---|---|---|---|
| Snails with oregano and shallots (page 106) | + | + | | + |
| Snails in a green sauce (page 106) | + | + | | + |

| Seafood | O | A | B | AB |
|---|---|---|---|---|
| Baked fish with shallots and ginger (page 108) | + | + | + | + |
| Cod steaks in yogurt and spices (page 109) | + | + | + | + |
| Gravlax (page 111) | + | + | + | + |
| Grilled tuna (page 112) | + | + | + | + |
| Marinated grilled tuna (page 113) | + | + | + | + |
| Monkfish en papillote (page 114) | + | + | + | + |
| Salmon mousse (page 115) | + | + | + | + |
| Salmon, lime and dill tartare (page 116) | + | + | + | + |

Wild sea bass (page 117)                            +   +

## Meat, Poultry and Game

|                                                      | O | A | B | AB |
|------------------------------------------------------|---|---|---|----|
| Braised beef (page 119)                              | + |   |   |    |
| Braised lamb with onions and lemons (page 120)       | + |   | + | +  |
| Marinated shoulder of lamb (page 121)                | + |   | + | +  |
| Our osso buco (page 122)                             | + |   | + |    |
| Steak tartare (page 123)                             | + |   | + |    |
| Chicken with preserved lemons (page 124)             | + | + |   |    |
| Chicken with tarragon (page 125)                     | + | + |   |    |
| Chicken with lemon, sage and garlic (page 126)       | + | + |   |    |
| Guinea fowl with sage (page 127)                     | + | + |   |    |
| Roast venison (page 128)                             | + |   | + |    |
| Marinated roast venison (page 129)                   | + |   | + |    |
| Ostrich steaks with shallots and red wine (page 130) | + | + | + | +  |
| Rabbit with preserved lemons (page 130)              | + |   | + | +  |
| Rabbit with provençale herbs (page 131)              | + |   | + | +  |
| Wild duck (page 132)                                 | + |   |   |    |

## Tofu and Tempeh

|                                                               | O | A | B | AB |
|---------------------------------------------------------------|---|---|---|----|
| Marinated tofu brochettes with thyme and oregano (page 134)   | + | + |   | +  |
| Marinated tempeh (page 135)                                   | + | + |   | +  |
| Marinated tofu (page 135)                                     | + | + |   | +  |
| Pan-fried tempeh (page 136)                                   | + | + |   | +  |

## Sauces

|                                      | O | A | B | AB |
|--------------------------------------|---|---|---|----|
| Aïoli (page 138)                     | + | + | + | +  |
| Fresh coriander sauce (page 139)     | + | + | + | +  |
| Ginger and tamari sauce (page 140)   | + | + | + | +  |
| Parsley sauce (page 141)             | + | + | + | +  |
| Soya yogurt dill sauce (page 142)    | + | + |   | +  |
| Summer salad dressing (page 142)     | + | + | + | +  |
| Sweet basil sauce (page 143)         | + | + | + | +  |
| Vinaigrette dressing (page 144)      | + | + | + | +  |

## Desserts

|                                                  | O | A | B | AB |
|--------------------------------------------------|---|---|---|----|
| Apple, walnut and maple syrup pie (page 147)     |   |   | + |    |
| Autumn apple pie (page 148)                      | + | + |   |    |
| Chocolate delight (page 149)                     | + | + |   | +  |
| Dark plum pie (page 150)                         | + | + | + | +  |
| Pear fruit salad (page 151)                      | + | + | + | +  |
| Plum crumble (page 152)                          | + | + | + | +  |

# bibliography

*Eat Right for Your Type*, Dr Peter J. D'Adamo, published by Putnam, 1996

*Cook Right For Your Type*, Dr Peter J. D'Adamo, published by Putnam, 1998

*Live Right for Your Type*, Dr Peter J. D'Adamo, published by Putnam, 2001

*The Encyclopedia of Medicinal Plants*, Andrew Chevallier, published by Dorling Kindersley, 1996

*The Diet Cure*, Julia Ross, published by Michael Joseph, 2000

*Culinary Herbs* by Ernest Small, issued by The National Research Council of Canada, 1997

*Fats That Heal, Fats That Kill*, Udo Erasmus, published in Canada by Alive Books, 1993

*The Healing Power of Foods*, Michael T. Murray, published in US by Prima Publishing, 1993

*The Healing Power of Herbs*, Michael T. Murray, published in US by Prima Publishing, 1995

*The Food Pharmacy*, Jean Carper, published by Positive Paperbacks, Simon & Schuster, 1990

*Food Your Miracle Medicine*, Jean Carper, published in US by Harper Perennial, 1994

*The Miracle Heart*, Jean Carper, published in US by Harper Paperbacks, 2000

*The Complete Book of Enzyme Therapy*, Dr Anthony J Cichoke, published in US by Avery, 1999

*Optimal Wellness*, Dr Ralph Golan, published in US by Ballantine Books, 1995

*Protein Power*, Drs Michael and Mary Dan Eades, published in US by Bantam, 1996

*Mastering the Zone*, Barry Sears, PhD, published by HarperCollins, 1997

*Raw Energy*, Leslie and Susannah Kenton, published by Vermillion, 1994

*The Plants we Need to Eat*, Jeannette Ewin, published by Thorsons, 1997

*Sugar and Your Health*, Ray C. Wunderlich, published in US by Good Health Publications, 1982

*Our Stolen Future*, Theo Colborn, Dianne Dumanosky and John Peterson Myers,
published in US by Dutton, 1996

*How To Live To Be 100*, Sula Benet, published in US by Dial Press, 1976

*The Liver Detox Plan*, Xandria Williams, published by Vermillion, 1998

*The Green Tea Book*, Lester A. Mitscher, PhD, published in US by Avery, 1998

*The Ginger Book*, Stephen Fulder, PhD, published in US by Avery, 1996

*The Way of Herbs*, Michael Tierra, published in US by Pocket Books (Simon & Schuster), 1998

*Herbs That Heal*, H. K. Bakhru, published in India by Orient Paperbacks, 1996

*Foods That Heal*, H. K. Bakhru, published in India by Orient Paperbacks, 1992

*Genetic Nutritioneering*, Jeffrey S. Bland, PhD, published in US by Keats, 1999

*Nourishing Traditions*, Sally Fallon, published in US by New Trends Publishing, 1999

*L'Ananas, "Roi des Fruits"*, Barbara Simonsohn, published in France by Librairie de Mèdicis, 2000

*Secrets D'une Herboriste*, Marie-Antoinette Mulot, published in France by Editions du Dauphin, 1999

*L'Aromatherapie*, Dr Jean Valnet, published in France by Maloine, 1990

*Au Bonheur des Plantes*, Michel Pierre et Michel Lis, published in France by Le Prè au Clercs, 1992.

# resources

The UK stockist of products related to the blood type diet (including multivitamins, multiminerals, probiotics, lectin blockers, test kits etc.) is:

Stacktheme Ltd
59 Bridge Street
Dollar FK14 7DQ
SCOTLAND
Tel: +44 (0) 1259 743255
Fax: +44 (0) 1259 743002
Email: Info@stacktheme.com

In the US contact:

North American Pharamacal Inc.
5 Brook Street
Norwalk, CT 06851
Tel: +1 203 866 7664
Fax: +1 203 838 4066
Email: www4yourtype.com

Dr D'Adamo's website can be found at: www.dadamo.com
This features complementary information not included in his books, as well as a list of nutritionists around the world who use the blood type diet.

# index